# Psychiatry, Politics and PTSD

Integrating critical and feminist psychology, psychiatry, and psychoanalysis, this text offers a distinct perspective on posttraumatic stress disorder (PTSD) as a clinical and social phenomenon.

The book draws upon interviews carried out in field settings to examine the true individual and social costs of being diagnosed with PTSD. The author examines how social contexts and social movements shape diagnostic thinking about mental trauma and how the PTSD diagnosis emerged as a symptom of a crisis in psychiatry over demands to recognize the social and political origins of mental suffering. Chapters explore case examples from a range of settings, such as military and veterans' affairs clinics, war zones and refugee camps, psychosomatic medicine, the criminal justice system, and more.

Providing a new way of thinking about PTSD and an alternative to both critics and defenders of the diagnosis, this text will be useful for scholars and practitioners in psychiatry, psychology, psychoanalysis and public health policy, as well as those in sociology, social work, gender studies, and the law.

**Janice Haaken, PhD**, is Professor Emeritus of Psychology at Portland State University, a Clinical Psychologist, and an award-winning documentary filmmaker.

"Janice Haaken is one of feminist critical psychology's most powerful voices. Here again, as in all her books and films, we discover that Haaken, a consummate storyteller, is also a consummate listener. The stories she tells here, drawn from her documentary film work and her clinical experience, reveal over and over the complexities of what it means to suffer and what it means to be human—complexities that defy any simple diagnosis. Haaken's capacity to hear in these stories what has too often been unheard illuminates for clinicians, activists, and social theorists alike the regressive and progressive socio-political uses—over its long history—of the PTSD diagnosis."

—**Lynne Layton, PhD**, Assistant Professor of Psychology, Department of Psychiatry, Harvard Medical School

"While not forgetting the suffering of real people, Haaken focuses on the way in which PTSD serves as a defense for those in the helping and healing professions. PTSD becomes a shape-shifting diagnosis, serving more to satisfy the needs of practitioners than the suffering of human beings. At the same time, the suffering designated by the diagnosis of PTSD is real and important. Haaken's ability to see PTSD both as an expression of the culture of the mental health profession, as well as an expression of deep human suffering, is unparalleled. This is a remarkable book by a remarkable author; psychoanalytic therapist, professor, scholar, and documentary filmmaker embedded in a Combat Stress Control unit in Afghanistan. No other book brings this wide-ranging and up-close access to the politics and experience of PTSD. No other book combines scholarship with experience in this way. A remarkable achievement."

—**Fred Alford, PhD**, Professor Emeritus, University of Maryland, College Park

"In her new book, Janice Haaken once again comes to our aid by examining and critically interpreting another of psychology's sacred cows. This time she studies the psychiatric diagnosis PTSD, a remarkably popular concept in pop culture and everyday language as well as professional therapeutic circles. But what are its political functions and moral meanings? With her characteristically lucid prose and critical intellectual gifts, Janice Haaken interprets PTSD through the lenses of politics, history, and feminist psychoanalysis. She sheds light on how PTSD has emerged and grown powerful as a diagnosis and how it serves not only to help patients but also to protect clinicians and limit their understandings of how and why patients suffer. Importantly, she accomplishes this with compassion, fairness, and clinical acumen; she sees many sides of the same problem and never loses sight of the people who suffer and those who are tasked with attenuating that suffering. Above all, she demonstrates how the psy disciplines could be a force for good by drawing on critical traditions and contributing to forms of resistance against the status quo. *Psychiatry, Politics and PTSD* is a book to be savored both by psy practitioners and general intellectual audiences throughout the world."

**—Philip Cushman, PhD**, retired core faculty,
Antioch University Seattle

"This book is essential reading. It's a superb, scholarly, timely and inspiring work that brings together a lifetime's critical analysis of psychiatry and the politics of posttraumatic stress disorder, using biographical, filmic, visual, participatory and field-based research. Important lines of analyses include the societal aspects of mental suffering, moral discourse on criminality, and the use of personality disorder and PTSD diagnoses as they underpin the social project of psychiatry. This book will be on my core reading lists for sociology, women's studies, critical and cultural criminology."

**—Maggie O'Neill, PhD**, Professor of Sociology
and Criminology, University College Cork

"This pathbreaking and invaluable book breaks down psychiatric conceptions of PTSD, reconstructing the history of the diagnostic category through a critical feminist psychoanalytic lens, and documents its functions in military contexts. Haaken's historical analysis and critique artfully bridge the worlds of theory and a range of practices, from clinical settings, war zones, the courts and crisis work, to political activism."

**—Ian Parker, PhD**, Practicing Psychoanalyst; Secretary,
Manchester Psychoanalytic Matrix

# Psychiatry, Politics and PTSD

## Breaking Down

Janice Haaken

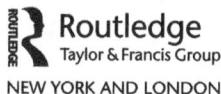

Routledge
Taylor & Francis Group

NEW YORK AND LONDON

First published 2021
by Routledge
52 Vanderbilt Avenue, New York, NY 10017

and by Routledge
2 Park Square, Milton Park, Abingdon, Oxon, OX14 4RN

*Routledge is an imprint of the Taylor & Francis Group, an informa business*

*Library of Congress Cataloging-in-Publication Data*
Names: Haaken, Jan, author.
Title: Psychiatry, politics and PTSD : breaking down / Janice Haaken.
Description: New York, NY : Routledge, 2020. | Includes bibliographical references and index.
Identifiers: LCCN 2020010558 (print) | LCCN 2020010559 (ebook) | ISBN 9780367819385 (hardback) | ISBN 9780367819378 (paperback) | ISBN 9781003010913 (ebook)
Subjects: LCSH: Post-traumatic stress disorder. | Post-traumatic stress disorder—Political aspects. | Feminist therapy. | Post traumatic stress disorder—Social aspects. | Post-traumatic stress disorder—Case studies.
Classification: LCC RC552.P67 H32 2020 (print) | LCC RC552.P67 (ebook) | DDC 616.85/21—dc23
LC record available at https://lccn.loc.gov/2020010558
LC ebook record available at https://lccn.loc.gov/2020010559

ISBN: 978-0-367-81938-5 (hbk)
ISBN: 978-0-367-81937-8 (pbk)
ISBN: 978-1-003-01091-3 (ebk)

Typeset in Times New Roman
by Apex CoVantage, LLC

# Contents

# Acknowledgments

This book grew out of participatory action research and documentary films carried out in crisis settings over a number of years, from refugee camps, war zones, protest encampments, military and VA hospitals, domestic violence shelters and prisons to state psychiatric hospitals. These projects required thinking through my ethical obligations to people in vulnerable situations, both staff members and those who identified as refugees, patients, clients, soldiers, or prisoners. Legal guidelines for carrying out interviews in many of these sites involved following HIPPA (Health Insurance Portability and Accountability Act) guidelines. In addition to protecting the rights to privacy and confidentiality in health settings, HIPPA recognizes the rights of patients to speak to media and scholars. In filming at the Oregon State Hospital, for example, patients invited to participate met with their attorneys to establish that they understood the educational nature of the documentary and that they were capable of consenting to public use of their stories. Many of the principles that guide my participatory action research (PAR) were carried into my documentary filmmaking—methods that enlist subjects/participants in generating key questions to be pursued, offering comments on work samples, and participating in panels at conferences or Q and A sessions after screenings. A key principle guiding this work is that marginalized people hold important insights on the world around them and on the broader society. This participatory tradition of inquiry stresses knowledge produced on the social margins and through various forms of human struggle.

For the many participants who shared their stories and insights, I am deeply grateful. This book is a culmination of my effort to bring lesser known perspectives on emotional suffering into the literature on posttraumatic stress disorder. In addition to expressing my gratitude to these participants, I want to thank the many clinicians working in crisis zones who shared their own experiences. I hope that I have done justice to the enormous challenges they face in helping people in difficult situations.

Over my career as a professor of psychology at Portland State University, I have had the joy of working with colleagues and students who share my passion for going beyond the walls of the university into difficult field settings and for producing knowledge that contributes to an emancipatory vision of society. Graduate and post-baccalaureate students on my field research and documentary teams include Diana Rempe, Jimena Alvarado, Jen Wallin-Ruschman, Tessa Palmer, Marial Stadick, Joseph Van der Naald, Darryl James, Bayard Lyons, and Samantha Praus. As one of my graduate students who later became a close colleague in the field of peace studies, Ariel Ladum contributed to work cited here as well as providing editorial assistance. I also want to thank my generous colleagues who read and commented on earlier versions: Patricia Kullberg for her astute comments at numerous stages of the manuscript; Johanna Brenner and Sherwin Davidson for insightful feedback at writing retreats and through their close readings of various chapters; Chris Lowe for consultations on the thesis of the book; Fred Alford for his encouragement and advice on the structuring of the manuscript; Marta Greenwald for discussions on ethical dilemmas in field research; and my partner, Tom Becker, for his boundless support and his many editorial and intellectual contributions throughout the writing process. And I want to thank my son and fellow filmmaker, Caleb Heymann, who helped to conceptualize and carry out my documentary projects, as well as fellow filmmaker and friend Eric Edwards. Both of these cinematographers brought their craftmanship, generosity, and deep sensitivity to the people and to the places where the projects were carried out.

I wish to express a special gratitude to Gary Mac Smith, an artist, psychotherapist and psychiatrist, for permitting the use of one of his paintings on the cover of this book, and for his keen observational skills as a clinician and a painter.

And, finally, I want to recognize my dear friend and colleague Tod (Theo) Sloan, who died in 2018. We shared a love for critical traditions in psychology and for bringing psychoanalysis into the joys and sorrows of activism, and to the difficult work of imagining that a better world is possible.

*The insoluble conflict between the claims of humanity, which normally carry decisive weight for a physician, and the demands of a national war was bound to confuse his activity.*

—Sigmund Freud, 1920

# Introduction

The subtitle of this book, *Breaking Down*, invokes an old idea in Western culture—the sudden development of a "nervous breakdown," a situation spoken of in hushed tones in my youth as a member of a Christian fundamentalist community. A number of the women in our church suffered such conditions—a label that carried a mix of sympathy and shame. The congregation's diagnosis of these church ladies—the "shut-ins" so notably out of sight at the Sunday morning church service—also conveyed hesitation in identifying the congregant as deviant. Whereas sinners bore responsibility for yielding to the influence of the devil, those suffering from nervous breakdowns occupied a more ambiguous place in our religious fold. Whether a housewife who kept her blinds closed all day or the old man staring blankly at no particular object, those suffering from nervous breakdowns warranted our pity and our prayers.

Posttraumatic stress disorder is heir to that old idiom of the nervous breakdown because it similarly captures a wide swath of troubles that summon public sympathies. The indicators of PTSD include symptoms of anxiety, memory disturbances, intrusive thoughts, problems in regulating mood and interpersonal relationships, and loss or decline in functioning (Levin, Kleinman, & Adler, 2014; Levy, 1995; Richardson, Sareen, Stein, & Ovuga, 2012; Scott, 1990). Since PTSD symptoms overlap considerably with related mental conditions, the diagnosis depends most crucially on identifying a traumatic event as cause of the clinical syndrome. As an idiom of everyday distress, PTSD offers a shorthand explanation for emotionally powerful scenes from the past that intrude on the present. At this level of popular usage, the broad reach of this relatively destigmatized disorder becomes a non-specific modern way of saying, "You are having a nervous breakdown."

The path of the PTSD diagnosis through the procedural rules of psychiatry tells a different story, however. All psychiatric diagnoses fail to capture the complex, dynamic, contextual, and idiosyncratic nature of human troubles. But PTSD departs from many of the hundreds of other categories available to clinicians in its recognition of societal causes of suffering, for example, warfare and sexual assault. The anti-psychiatry movement of the 1960s and 1970s, along with the anti-war and feminist movements, took aim at psychiatry for its failure to address political factors in the development of clinical syndromes and for its collusion in the very problems that the profession claims to alleviate. But as the PTSD diagnosis gained official recognition, it became symptomatic of a deeper crisis in psychiatry over its role in the social management of suffering.

*Psychiatry, Politics and PTSD* draws on over 200 interviews carried out in field settings—in war zones, psychiatric hospitals, and refugee camps. Most of the stories included in the book are based on interviews with clinicians whose job it is to help people in terrible situations. These are also situations where institutions have assumed responsibility for some aspect of the care of afflicted people, whether veterans, persons hospitalized for crimes, or refugees. I include a number of stories of people in the role of patients as well and integrate their insights on the various diagnoses assigned to them. Participants have agreed to this public use of their accounts.

The chapters in the book are organized around sites of intense controversy over PTSD as a way of framing the problems of people, from the use of the diagnosis in legal settings, war zones, medical conditions, and disability claims, to various global conflict zones. This introduction lays out key concepts and theoretical frameworks guiding the inquiry and my main lines of analysis pursued throughout the book.

## Psychic Trauma

The concept of psychic trauma holds a deep place—some would say a sacred place—in the history of psychology. Whether invoked in scholarly conferences or everyday discourse, the term calls for a careful mode of listening. Unlike physical trauma, the impacts of emotional trauma are more elusive. They require some capacity to visualize the unseen, like shadowy figures in the dark. Yet this metaphor of hiddenness, regularly invoked in the trauma literature, should invite scrutiny of the tools through which the concealed is revealed. I have previously written about those tools and their limits, including the tools of my own psychoanalytic practices (1998, 2010).

In the various arenas where I have worked as a psychologist—from field research, psychotherapy, teaching, and documentary filmmaking, to political activism—trauma stories have captured my imagination as well as my scholarly interest. Traumatic experiences are often described as beyond words, as events that overtake the psyche. Over the course of my career as a clinician, I have helped people to put painful parts of their histories into words. But most of my field research and documentaries have focused on the professionals whose job it is to assist people in this same process.

Literary critic and trauma theorist Cathy Caruth (2014) positions the therapist as mediator between the fragmented and emotionally charged imagery associated with trauma and representations of events in the form of a memory or testimonial: "It's [trauma] all forming itself or being reconstructed, recreated in the symbolizing process of the therapist" (p. 17). The "talking cure"—the term used early on to describe psychoanalysis—remains a cornerstone of clinical practice. But the talking cure involves listening with "a third ear"— attending to communicative gaps, to silences, to the multiple meanings accompanying mental disturbances.

Listening with a third ear means lingering in situations of uncertainty and avoiding premature interpretations. While biological psychiatry aims to control or eliminate the symptom, psychoanalysis from Freud on has taken up the idea that the symptom tells a story—and that the subjective responses of the clinician enter into the translation of that story. Shoshana Felman (1992) offers that psychoanalysis requires attentiveness to the anxieties and defenses that professional listeners bring to the clinical encounter. She makes the case that the revolutionary potential of psychoanalysis lies in its relational approach to truth, the idea that "it takes two to witness the unconscious" (p. 15). Felman goes on to extend the reach of psychoanalysis into the public sphere: "Psychoanalysis, in this way, profoundly rethinks and radically renews the very concept of testimony . . . that the speaking subject constantly bears witness to a truth that nonetheless continues to escape him" (p. 15). This vision of a radical psychoanalysis calls for considerable humility and care in how we make use of the tools of our trade.

In this book, I turn my third ear toward palpable tensions in the profession of psychiatry, and particularly to how PTSD acquired its status as a politically progressive diagnosis. Through my historical analysis and field interviews, I make the argument that the diagnosis grew out of pressures on psychiatry that threatened its legitimacy. PTSD acquired socially symbolic currencies over time as a label that seemed to have transcended the prejudices of earlier diagnoses, for example, hysteria and psychopathy. In field research carried out over 20 years, I became interested in how practitioners were enlisting the PTSD category as a way of managing seemingly impossible clinical tasks—situations where they were negotiating various institutional, political, and psychological demands. And I began to focus on how the diagnosis itself served as a defensive coping strategy for clinicians.

In Western societies, psychologists and psychiatrists have played leading roles over the past century in interpreting stress conditions. Much of this work has been carried out in the context of warfare—a primary site for the psychological study and treatment of mental breakdown under conditions of extreme pressure. My own profession of psychology carries a long and deep history of involvement in warfare and post-war treatment of veterans—history taken up at various junctures in this book. Largely overlooked in my profession's vast literature on stress and trauma conditions associated with warfare, however, is the role of *translators* on the scene—particularly clinicians—who take on the task of producing coherence out of the inchoate and fragmented images associated with trauma reactions. To the extent that translators are part of Felman's formula that it "takes two to witness the unconscious," assessments tend to hone in on problems related to denial or other distancing defenses (Felman, 1992, p. 15). The experience of being emotionally moved by the testimony tends to be endorsed as evidence of both its truth value and the therapeutic effectiveness of the exchange. As part of a roundtable on decolonizing trauma theory, Steph Craps and colleagues (2015) suggest that the field of "trauma studies has always been critical of detachment" and that "it is a basic assumption of much trauma theory that readers or viewers should be affected by trauma testimonies they read or view" (p. 915).

Many clinicians working in conflict zones describe their duty to "bear witness to trauma" in building a public record from the fragmented memories of direct survivors (Alford, 2009). Benjamin (2018) points out that "the experience of the failed witness is a central component of trauma" (p. 227). The trauma originates not only in the direct impact of an event but in the absence of a holding environment or modes of recognizing the harms suffered. This failure may take the form of abandoning victims or of "not seeing them as worth saving." But failures abound in many virtuous attempts to provide aid and recognition as well.

## Psychiatry and the Politics of Diagnosis

The story of PTSD is inextricably bound up in the politics of the *Diagnostic and Statistical Manual*—the DSM—which is often described as the bible of the mental health field. Many lay people are vaguely familiar with this tome, which catalogues an ever-expanding array of conditions and criteria. At different junctures in this book, the DSM enters my story of PTSD. With each revised edition, from DSM I in 1952 through DSM-5 in 2013, disagreements over the causes and definitions of mental disorders have been a source of pitched debate (Brewin, Lanius, Novac, Schnyder, & Galea, 2009; Probst, 2014; Stein et al., 2010). Psychoanalysis shaped the first two editions of the manual. But as psychoanalysis lost status in psychiatry, DSM committees jettisoned language associated with this legacy. They adopted a purely descriptive approach where disorders are identified by clusters of signs rather than inferences concerning underlying etiology (Wilson, 1993).

Cultural critic Sam Kriss (2013) describes the DSM-5 as a "book of lamentations," approaching the text as analogous to a novel. He offers that "we have an entire book, something that purports to be a kind of encyclopedia of madness, a Library of Babel for the mind, containing everything that can possibly be wrong with a human being" (para. 5). There is an affinity between the lamentation offered by Kriss and my own approach to psychiatric taxonomies. In characterizing the American Psychiatric Association, the author of the manual, Kriss comments sardonically that

> what the narrator of this story is describing is its own solitude, its own inability to appreciate other people, and its own overpowering desire

for death—but the real horror lies in the world that could produce such a voice.

(para. 17)

The American Psychiatric Association holds a controlling interest in the DSM project and its aim of producing a scientifically grounded taxonomy, as well as reaping the enormous revenues generated by its sale. But, like many religious texts, the DSM is rife with contradictions. Practitioners bring their own interpretations of its arcane truths to the messy world of human experience.

The introduction to DSM-5 acknowledges scientific support for fluidity across diagnostic categories. "The boundaries between many disorder 'categories' are more fluid over the life course than DSM-IV recognized, and many symptoms assigned to a single disorder may occur, at varying levels of severity, in many other disorders" (American Psychiatric Association, 2013, p. 5). The DSM-5 expands many diagnoses and their criteria while eliminating others. There are real consequences to these changes, in that a diagnosis is required for billable services in the health care system and for disability claims. All diagnoses involve translating stories of suffering into the categories available for making sense of that suffering. But PTSD has proven to be among the most resilient of the psychiatric diagnoses in surviving categorical purges within official psychiatry.

Critiques of psychiatry target its reliance on psychopharmacological remedies—an area that includes treatment for PTSD. But my interest in psychiatry centers on its powerful role in producing and regulating diagnostic categories. In the mental health field as a whole, psychotherapy and counseling remain the skills most associated with the relief of emotional suffering. Through its authorship of official diagnoses, the American Psychiatric Association and psychiatry as a medical specialty occupy a powerful place in the mental health field. Yet this power faces challenges and various crises of legitimacy, including within psychiatry itself. The book brings PTSD into this history of crises in the field of psychiatry and particularly in response to the social movements of the 1970s.

The definition of PTSD has changed over its history as a recognized psychiatric disorder—changes taken up in this book. But a cluster of symptoms continues as the core syndrome: The person experiences psychological and physiological reactions to a distressing event that endures beyond a culturally acceptable period of time. Considered normal and adaptive responses to threats, the reactions become a disorder when they persist long after the threat has passed. The concepts underpinning the diagnosis have remained relatively stable, as has the treatment aim of helping the person to achieve emotional distance from a disturbing scene from the past.

With the publication of DSM-III in 1980, many clinicians celebrated the entry of PTSD as an unequivocal marker of progress in acknowledging societal causes of mental disturbances (McHugh & Treisman, 2007; Scott, 1990).

In attributing a mental disorder to an external event, the diagnosis widened the legal space for many victims' claims as well. And its inclusion in the DSM-III led to reclassification of many previously stigmatized conditions and created new ways of looking at those conditions. As an early champion of the diagnosis, Jonathan Shay (1994), describes the history of mental health misrecognition of veterans' suffering:

> Combat veterans in our program who first made contact with the mental health system in the early 1970s were almost universally diagnosed as paranoid schizophrenic, if first seen in the late 1970s as manic-depressive or schizo-affective, and if first seen in the mid-1980s as suffering from PTSD.

He adds that the disorder "can unfortunately mimic virtually any condition in psychiatry" (p. 169). This progression from the most serious of the mental disorders to increasingly treatable diagnostic categories registered the trend toward normalizing myriad psychiatric symptoms as indicators of trauma. Seventeen psychiatric symptoms were listed in the DSM-III-R posttraumatic stress disorder criteria, with the primary criterion for differential diagnosis that "the person has experienced an event that is outside the range of usual human experience and that would be markedly distressing to almost anyone" (American Psychiatric Association, 1987, p. 287). Rather than the standard psychiatric script of a normal façade concealing a disturbed interior, with Dr. Jekyll slowly revealing the menacing Mr. Hyde, the PTSD profile brought to the stage the potential for madness in everyone.

Because the diagnosis requires establishing an impactful event as the cause of a symptom complex, the PTSD disorder inevitably raises questions about human memory as well. Irene Visser (2015) notes that the trauma field rests on a set of taken-for-granted metaphors. The memory trace, thought to be "implanted in the psyche," is further claimed to make "itself known through a series of symptoms" (p. 252). Many critics of the diagnosis point out that subjective judgments inevitably arise, including in establishing the causal status of the traumatic memory. Felicity Callard (2014) calls for thinking of diagnostic practices as a dynamic process where the meaning of events to the patient and the social contexts that shape their determinative power can shift over time. I show here how the obsessive tendency in psychiatry to "pin down" PTSD within a stable, trans-historical taxonomy is itself symptomatic of the anxiety associated with this diagnosis.

## Lines of Analysis

One line of analysis in this book centers on questions about the progressiveness of the PTSD diagnosis—the extent to which the category responds, beyond its military associations, to the grievances of groups historically marginalized, for example, women, racial and sexual minorities, the working class, and the poor. I explain how the diagnosis lost its progressive animus as it was incorporated into psychiatric taxonomies. This does not suggest that the diagnosis no longer holds instrumental value for groups or individuals. In popular discourse and clinical and legal settings, PTSD remains a diagnosis that provides the means for making claims on institutions and society for support. The book shows how the rules for making claims entail compromises—much like a neurosis itself represents a compromise between conflicting forces.

A second line of analysis explores the role of psychoanalysis in the PTSD movement. In *The Shattered Self* (Ulman & Brothers, 1988), psychoanalysts Richard Ulman and Doris Brothers urge therapists to "return to the trauma paradigm" as the early foundation of psychoanalytic thought. Leading psychiatrists in the trauma field in the late 20th century, notably Bessel van der Kolk (2015) and Alice Miller (2006), draw on psychoanalytic constructs in advancing the concept of body memory and lowering clinical thresholds for diagnosing signs of trauma. Yet the critical potential of psychoanalysis was blunted by its alliances with the trauma therapy movement and its problematic use of the concept of the unconscious. In looking back on the role of psychoanalysis in the PTSD movement, I explain how diagnostic premises of PTSD run counter to many psychoanalytic principles, and particularly the concept of over-determination—the idea that causal events in the life of a person inevitably carry the weight of prior histories.

A third analysis pursued here looks at how the political and historical contexts of stressful or traumatic events enter into diagnostic thinking. The early PTSD movement emphasized social arrangements that shape clinical reactions to traumatic events, for example, how the military hierarchy scapegoats those under their command in assigning responsibility for war atrocities after a firefight. But as advocates sought to shore up the legitimacy of PTSD within the diagnostic rules, their emphasis on the societal context receded. Fighting for entry into the DSM system meant establishing the universality of the condition and its fit with the medical model. The social history that unfolds here recognizes early PTSD advocates as part of mass movements challenging dominant institutions. Yet the legitimacy of the diagnosis required that the "extreme stressor" criterion departed from everyday experience. Even though everyone theoretically could develop PTSD as a "normal response to an abnormal situation," the claims of oppressed groups, including the poor and the incarcerated, often fell below the threshold criteria. For those suffering harms more diffusely located in history or based on more systematic forms of violence or neglect, for example, polluted neighborhoods or poorly run schools, the diagnosis failed as a register of their claims. PTSD required a dramatic story that raised the account above less riveting images of chronic misery. And it demanded a distinct and decisive origin in the past.

Because trauma has acquired moral status as a condition associated with abuse and violence, questions about the potential over-reach and rigidification of the PTSD diagnosis can seem insensitive. Vast resources are now invested in PTSD outcome research, and it is the second most common condition for awarding disability payments through the Veterans Administration (VA), the first being hearing loss (Frueh, Grubaugh, Elhai, & Buckley, 2007; Levin et al., 2014; McNally & Frueh, 2013). As a result, there are enormous stakes in both defending the legitimacy of the disorder and reducing costs. The focus here on the diagnosis as a symptom of conflict in the field of psychiatry is not meant to downplay the suffering of PTSD patients. Rather, the critique centers on how this diagnosis operates on an institutional level and how the criteria for diagnosis limits the kinds of stories that get told and modes of listening to those stories.

## Traumatic Stress: Working at the Hyphen

In deconstructing the diagnosis of PTSD, this book works at the conceptual borders between *stress* and *trauma*—terms thought to hold a natural affinity as operating in tandem along a continuum. For over a century, the United States government and private industry have supported research on human responses to stress, with much of this research guided by a mechanistic model of mind. People, like machines, are subject to breakdown under conditions that exceed their operational capacities. And maintenance of both people and machines requires identifying stress points and developing technologies and skills for their upkeep. As founder of industrial psychology John B. Watson (1925) once pronounced, the purpose of behavioral psychology is "to state what the human machine is good for and to render serviceable predictions about its future capacities whenever society needs such information" (p. 218). The military has called upon psychology for such information since World War I. Military behavioral health practitioners often describe soldiers as "assets," and the practitioner's job to be "force multipliers" in getting more out of these military assets (D. Rabb, personal communication, July 4, 2011). Stress research has tended to approach the human body as a bundle of mechanisms. It is largely an impersonal model of mind.

Trauma studies, on the other hand, tend to be more aligned with what we ordinarily think of as psychology—the subjective self and its processes of making sense of the world. The field of trauma studies holds a particular affinity with psychodynamic traditions in its focus on storytelling and mental representations of self and other. While trauma may refer to either an event or a response to an event, the term invites a narrative account of some kind. To speak of psychic trauma is to position the problem within a moral community of responsibility as well (Caruth, 1991; Laub, 2009). Whereas stress researchers produce observations based on biological markers of strain and breakdown in mental mechanisms, trauma researchers speak of the ethics of bearing witness to "wounds of the soul" or to an existential collapse in meaning (Bremner & Marmar, 2002; van der Kolk, 2015). Whereas stress speaks to the machinery of mind, trauma evokes images of the ghosts in those machines. The contemporary discourse on the "moral injuries of war" holds an affinity with this latter approach in invoking metaphors that frame trauma as a spiritual crisis (Nash & Litz, 2013).

What do these differing models communicate to us about the disorder of PTSD? Is one set of metaphors better than the other, or does each speak to some partial truth? In looking back on the history of how the stress and trauma psychologies joined forces, I explain how the union of these fields of study was tense from the very start. I show how the expansion of the PTSD diagnosis exposed—like a machine operating beyond its capacity—problems in the models cobbled together to advance the legitimacy of the diagnosis.

The military literature provides the best sources for studying PTSD as this stress-trauma condition. Military psychologists developed the first standardized measures for assessing how much pressure people could endure before breaking down. The Department of Defense and the VA Administration are also the places where people who break down have the strongest claims for reparations. Psychiatrist Norman Camp (2015), author of *US Army Psychiatry in the Vietnam War*, a military psychiatry textbook, describes the intense controversies within this sub-field of medicine during the last half of the Vietnam War. In his review of lessons to be learned from the Vietnam War, Camp argues that the psychiatric categories available to clinicians were woefully inadequate in explaining the complex and situational array of disturbances displayed by the troops. Camp also takes up the politics of diagnosis. He claims that psychiatrists were pressured to diagnose soldiers on a large-scale basis under various personality disorder labels—an intervention that relieved the military of responsibility for service members' problems because of the widely shared assumption that these disorders are deeply rooted character problems. Troop troubles in military service were routinely dismissed as personality defects and soldiers discharged dishonorably. Some of these troubles were indeed likely influenced by personality factors. But the political context made this avenue of exploration more of a tool for the military than a means of understanding the struggles of soldiers.

While his review only touches on PTSD, Camp (2015) suggests that the category of PTSD obfuscates the complex dynamics of emotional reactions to warfare, just as did the use of the personality disorders: "Although the PTSD concept drew much needed medical attention to the treatment needs of Vietnam veterans, it simultaneously served to discredit veteran complaints of contributory mistreatment by society, the government, and the military" (p. 446). In my review, I explain how the concept of *moral injury* has entered into this same contested terrain. The growing literature on moral injury holds appeal for many progressive clinicians because it seems to explain the existential aspects of PTSD and to provide a corrective to the narrow criteria of the medical model.

My uneasiness with the expansion of PTSD preceded my venture into documenting military combat stress control in my film *Mind Zone: Therapists*

*Behind the Frontlines* (Haaken, 2014). But making this documentary brought me to the front lines of PTSD diagnostic practices. With the authorization of the United States Army, my crew and I were allowed to embed with a Combat Stress Control (CSC) medical detachment through their training and deployment to Afghanistan. It was one of many stress control teams mobilized during the peak of the US-led wars in Iraq and Afghanistan. This field project took me deeper into the tangled historical roots of this diagnosis in the business of warfare. A curious phenomenon took hold as the documentary entered the final phase of production and gathered media interest. Although the film explored a range of mental reactions of soldiers in war zones, for example, anxiety, depression, insomnia, and psychotic reactions, *Mind Zone* was typically described by the media as a film about troops and PTSD. Since many diagnoses overlap considerably with criteria for PTSD (Breslau, 2004; Dobbs, 2009; Frueh, Hamner, Cahill, Gold, & Hamlin, 2000; McHugh & Treisman, 2007; Orsillo et al., 1996; Summerfield, 2001), the category became the discursive container for a broad range of troubles associated with military service. Indeed, the story that had taken hold in the media in response to public anxieties over repeated deployments in the wars in Iraq and Afghanistan centered nearly exclusively on PTSD. Even suicide among veterans, associated with veterans' higher rate of access to weapons and depressive reactions, was framed as an outcome of untreated PTSD. The disorder had become the dominant lens through which mental reactions to warfare were viewed. I became increasingly curious about this cultural Rorschach card. Whatever the profile of distress that emerged in public discourse, the picture seemed to take the shape of a PTSD profile.

## The Anti-Psychiatry Movement

My first encounter with military trauma was in the context of resistance in the early 1970s to the Vietnam War, a time when I worked as a young psychiatric nurse at the University Hospital in Seattle and became captivated by the anti-psychiatry movement—a loose collection of intellectual and political projects focused on challenging the societal basis of psychiatric authority. Some rejected terms such as *treatment* and *patient* because of their affinity with biological models of illness. Many of the clinicians in the anti-psychiatry movement of the 1960s and 1970s were themselves psychiatrists and psychologists, as well as social workers, psychiatric nurses, and assistants working in mental health centers (Berlim & Fleck, 2003; Nasser, 1995; Sedgwick, 1982). Much of the therapeutic work was carried out in store-front clinics, and a great deal of this "street psychiatry" was organized around opposition to the Vietnam War.

What struck me as a young nurse in listening to anti-war veterans' groups was their feelings of betrayal by the military itself and their sense of moral obligation to oppose an unjust and irrational war. Many of these activist

Vietnam War veterans were so distrustful of the VA mental health system that they agitated for (and won) funding for Vet Centers with counseling services operating separate from the VA (Cheney et al., 2018; Cors, Lau, & Farmer, 2013; Isaacs, 2000; Macpherson, 1981). As much as these Centers provided treatment, they also operated as sites of solidarity and resistance to military-authorized accounts of their war-time experiences.

Marxist psychiatrists of that era, such as the South African psychoanalyst David Cooper (1990), developed analyses of psychiatric hospitals as part of the state apparatus for political control of groups cast as deviant. Peter Sedgwick (1982), a leading theorist in the anti-psychiatry movement, also contributed to this line of critique. But Sedgwick emphasized as well the progressive currents in modern psychiatry. He notes that the idiom of mental illness, no less than physical illness, registers distress and a claim on the culture for some form of care, whether through folk remedies or Western methods. Anti-psychiatry theorists often approach mental suffering from too much distance, Sedgwick contends, rather than from the "hard seat of the waiting room or the casualty department's stretcher" (p. 28). In arguing for patients' rights to care within the framework of health and social welfare, Sedgwick cautions against over-politicizing or romanticizing mental disorders. In the anti-psychiatry movement of the 1960s and 1970s, schizophrenia was embraced as the prototypical madness that spoke to the insanity of the larger social order. While delusions, hallucinations, and disordered thinking were recognized as signs of mental illness, these signs also spoke to the human condition more generally—a concept taken into the psychedelic movement of that same era.

Clinical interest in patients' experiences of hallucinations and delusions had faded by the 1980s. If psychotic people had anything to say, few in the mental health field were listening beyond the time it took to get them on meds. Trauma conditions were distinguished from severe mental illness and recouped some of the ground lost to the medicalization of madness—a development that I have described elsewhere (Haaken, 1998). Trauma treatment centered on extended periods of listening to disordered minds and accessing buried memories of horrific events (Cohen, 1993; Noble, 1993; Woollard, 1993). The hospital beds of long-term psychiatric facilities, once occupied by people diagnosed with major depression or schizophrenia, were by the 1990s reserved for trauma treatment.

Women were part of the anti-psychiatry movement of the 1970s even though men were the leading theorists (Proctor, 2018). A wave of feminist writings, from Phyllis Chesler's (1997) *Women and Madness* to Jerome Agel (1971) and other contributors to *The Radical Therapist Collective*, took aim at psychiatry and called for women to get off the analyst's couch and refuse the position of patient. For the middle-class white women who were finding their voice during the Second-wave, feminism meant rejecting the patriarchal idea of an inherent female vulnerability, refusing to see ourselves as "damaged goods" after rape or incest. Third-wave feminism—a movement that emerged in the 1990s and challenged many of the assumptions of the Second-wave—showed how narratives of injured womanhood circulated through the dialects of race and class (Haaken, 2016). Black women were more apt to be cast as indestructible than as inherently vulnerable (Collins, 2000; hooks, 1992). Trauma was a motif in many stories of female resistance, whether in consciousness-raising groups on domestic violence or speak-outs on rape and other forms of violence against women. But psychological trauma was not central to feminist discourse in that period. Casting off patriarchy meant confronting your oppressor while refusing the position of the damaged one.

By the 1990s, however, trauma had moved from the margins to the center of feminist campaigns, particularly in confronting child sexual abuse and recovering memories of early sexual abuse (see Ulman & Brothers, 1988). Women were being diagnosed with multiple personality disorder (MPD) in alarming numbers in the 1990s, a dramatic condition thought to be a female variant of PTSD. Trauma theorists claimed that these were essentially the same disorders with differing clinical pictures, with each being a response to overwhelming psychic shock (Ross, 1989; van der Kolk, 2015). Unlike other disorders associated with women historically, such as hysteria and borderline personality disorder, the language of the multiple acquired a heroic dignity. While the symptoms of the PTSD patient spoke of horrors on the battlefield, the dissociated states of the multiple expressed nightmares on the home front. Therapists played leading roles in excavating the hidden personalities thought to lie dormant in the psyche, naming the alters that emerged from these disturbing reports from the past. As therapists specializing in MPD uncovered an expanding cast of hidden personalities in female patients, each carrying increasingly gothic tales of early sexual violations, critics suspected that therapists were unconsciously directing these dramatic performances (Ganaway, 1989; Haaken, 1998)

My reading of the history of PTSD finds points of correspondence with the analysis of PTSD developed by Alan Young (1997) in *Harmony of Illusions: Inventing Post-Traumatic Stress Disorder*. He critiques the conventional psychiatric narrative that lists shell shock and the war neuroses as precursors to the modern discovery of PTSD—a narrative that casts practitioners of eras past as either misreading the signs or lacking the scientific tools to understand and treat the condition effectively. Young deconstructs this history, explaining how the legacy of PTSD reveals more about the expansion of biological psychiatry than it does psychiatric progress in responding to emotional suffering. He describes how the diagnosis increasingly relied on biological models of stress as PTSD researchers sought to enlist neurobiology and neuroendocrinology to advance its validity. "To obtain facts and findings," Young astutely concludes, "researchers now interrogate blood and urine rather than men" (p. 283). Young studied clinical interactions on a VA psychiatric unit after the Vietnam War, describing a quasi-religious belief in the PTSD model shared by clinicians and patients alike. After the liberalizing of criteria for making the diagnosis in the early 1990s, Young documents what he sees as a worrisome rise in Vietnam-era disability claims: "No one is left out in the cold; no one will forfeit a service-connected pension because of these changes" (p. 290). A growing chorus of critics sounds this same alarm today, including some of the early researchers who brought the diagnosis into the DSM-III in 1980 (McNally & Frueh, 2013).

The story of PTSD told here traces the development of some of these same concerns about over-use of the diagnosis and the politics of the PTSD movement. But I take the position that social constructionists such as Young leave too much of the PTSD phenomenon behind. Interesting questions concerning the role of psychiatry in framing human suffering are left unanswered. Disorders can be both socially constructed—as Young argues in the case of PTSD— and at the same time valid ways of understanding mental functioning. John B. Watson—discussed earlier in the context of a machine model of mind—placed psychology in the service of society. But his conception of what makes psychology serviceable was bound to a capitalist worldview—a view of human labor as a commodity to be maximized in a system of economic exchange. Few textbooks today offer such baldly instrumentalist views of psychology as a discipline. But powerful institutions, from pharmaceutical companies, health care institutions, and the American Psychiatric Association, to the US Department of Defense, continue to guide mental health knowledge and practices in ways that marginalize critical perspectives (Cushman, 2002, 2012).

While agreeing with some of the arguments of PTSD critics, I show how many of the criticisms focus too narrowly on the diagnosis as a "category crisis" rather than on the deeper dilemmas at the heart of this diagnosis and what it registers about the field of psychiatry itself. In my university courses on psychopathology, I often use PTSD as an exemplar of a condition that tells us more about the gains of mental health experts than it does the suffering of diagnosed individuals. PTSD has decisive appeal over a term such as hysteria, associated with Freudian old-school thinking, and it has survived the scandals that led to the taxonomic death of multiple personality disorder— also described as a trauma condition. PTSD is a "good diagnosis" because it establishes that even very normal people can look or act crazy under the right conditions, and its symptoms allow claims for support. The field of psychiatry itself is among those claimants.

## Diagnostic Storytelling

As a clinician, I am listening for the beginnings and endings of stories, places where the stage is set for other protagonists in the person's life situation and where potential resolutions to life's conflicts are staged. Freud introduced the concept of over-determination in interpreting the clinical significance of stories—how multiple factors contribute to the psychological meaning of events. Further, the beginning of a story may operate as a "screen memory" in protecting against more disturbing recollections (Freud, 1899/1962). From this perspective, the search for a determinative source of the patient's symptoms in past events confronts the shifting dynamics of mental life, from memory itself to motivational states and contexts that shape mental pictures of the past.

There is by now a PTSD genre of stories, and many of them run counter to psychoanalytic ways of thinking about diagnosis. From a psychoanalytic perspective, stories about others are in part stories about the self—with other protagonists in the drama sometimes registering unconscious aspects of the storyteller's own internal world. Victims' stories about abusers may represent both an objective threat and a conflict originating in the past that continues to occupy an important place in their psyches. A woman may protect her abuser not only because she relies on him for material support but because he represents a part of her own internal world—for example, what is experienced as a threatening internal object or aspect of her own desires (Benjamin, 1988, 2018). Cultural and historical contexts also structure how events are interpreted, including how boundaries between goodness and badness are drawn.

Clinicians are ethically required to take clients' cultural beliefs into account, including beliefs about emotional suffering. Yet cultural beliefs are not static or monolithic. Over time, the homophobic parent can become supportive in response to an adult child coming out of the closet. But relinquishing prejudices and the tales told to support them requires new stories with better endings. The parent of a gay or lesbian child in America today has more positive scripts available in thinking about that child's future than in previous decades when scripts were near uniformly tragic. The ethical obligation for clinicians is not to simply validate a belief because it is deeply rooted in a culture. In working with people that have suffered collective trauma or have been denied parts of their own identities, therapists do have a special obligation to listen longer and to reflect on personal blind spots.

The mental health field is itself a culture. In this book, I approach the PTSD diagnosis as a story circulating through the rituals and practices of the helping professions. One of the deepest organizing principles of a culture centers on concepts of time. The expectations laid out in the DSM guidelines for how long a person normally grieves before becoming clinically depressed, how long a person should be shaken by a car accident before being diagnosed with acute traumatic stress, how long a person rejected by a friend should be able to ruminate before developing an obsessive condition—all of these judgments along a continuum of normal to abnormal are based on cultural codes. The PTSD diagnostician enters into these codes and into the creation of a proscriptive denouement to the story of distress. My own training as a psychoanalytic clinician cautions against premature denouements. But there are material conditions in the delivery of mental health services—as well as in the society as a whole—that contribute to this press for closure. If you have to return to work after the loss of a loved one, the diagnosis of a grief reaction can be part of how the medical profession gets you back on your feet.

Through my work with refugees and immigrants in the United States and abroad, I have been sensitized to the problematic freight attached to exports of

Western psychiatry and to its obsession with taxonomies. Many of the women I have worked with in war zones reject the term posttraumatic stress disorder in describing the scenes of suffering that haunt their memories as survivors. Researchers and clinicians working internationally are often acutely aware of pitfalls in assigning Western categories to suffering in conflict zones (Kintsch & Greene, 1978; Lewis-Fernández & Kleinman, 1995; Mezzich et al., 1999; Shoeb, Weinstein, & Mollica, 2007). But the problem is often conceptualized as a conflict between "individualist" and "collectivist" models of suffering. Psychiatry is associated with the individualist frame, whereas many societies think in terms of group or familial frames of reference. While not without merit, this typology vastly over-simplifies cultural differences. Both Western and non-Western societies include recognition of bounded individuals—persons recognized by their unique features—as well as group identities. So too, traditional healers are often quite knowledgeable about Western notions of trauma, some of which are incorporated into their native practices (Eghigian, 2010). This is quite different from individualism as an ideology—a worldview that guides much of the field of psychiatry (Parker, 2013, 2015).

In situations of collective trauma, concerns more often center on how history is remembered and how responsibility for suffering is socially distributed rather on which people meet diagnostic criteria for a disorder (Shaw, 2007, 2012). Trauma invites a dramatic story centered on victims, perpetrators, and rescuers. Psychiatric diagnoses tend to narrow the stage for these dramas and to choreograph them in ways that conform to the profession's own protocols (Berrios, 1999; Cohen, 1993; Kleinman, 2012; Power, 2015). In many sites of conflict around the world, mental trauma is best understood in the context of political grievances. The clinical privatizing of stories of suffering, while potentially helpful to individuals, carries a heavy freight when applied to the experiences of people suffering as a group. Separating those in the group whose symptoms cross a clinical threshold is itself a problematic intervention in many such contexts. In this book, I show how this tendency of psychiatry to hyper-individualize and privatize suffering is problematic in the Western world/Northern hemisphere as well.

## Structure of the Book

The five chapters are organized around sites of intense conflict in the social history of PTSD—sites that have shaped the status and legitimacy of this diagnosis. Much like a patient's unfolding story and shifting accounts of events, the story of psychiatry, politics, and PTSD lends itself to multiple starting points. There is no decisive beginning, middle, or end. My account draws on my own participation in this history—my position as a practicing psychoanalytic clinician, a critical psychologist engaged in analysis of the societal contexts that shape my profession, and my work as a documentarian and field researcher interviewing other practitioners in crisis settings. I start with a series of clinical encounters—settings where people are talking with professionals about their troubles and some of the options available to clinicians in explaining them. The chapters unfold as they widen into sites where the PTSD diagnosis is introduced as a means of adjudicating various claims, from medical, legal/forensic, and disability cases to social justice movements.

The first chapter, "Listening to Distressing Stories," starts with how the PTSD narrative emerged as a call for a new mode of clinical listening. The focus on war stories in this chapter foregrounds how military institutions have profoundly shaped the PTSD criteria because warfare has long been associated with psychic trauma as well as human reactions to extreme stress. I present the case of a veteran diagnosed with PTSD who I interviewed a number of times over a period of a year. The case foregrounds junctures in his story that open differing interpretive possibilities and a rationale for returning to the abandoned diagnosis of war neurosis. The chapter includes military sexual trauma (MST)—a sub-genre of PTSD that gained wide currency in the 2000s—and addresses the constraints for female veterans as they enlist this version of the PTSD story.

Chapter 2, "Trauma and Troubled Personalities," takes up conditions where PTSD advocates have expanded the disorder into the taxonomic terrain of the personality disorders—an area where psychiatry confronts some of its most trenchant political criticisms. Termed Axis II conditions prior to the DSM-5, these disorders are thought to be highly resistant to treatment. Their use by military doctors has also been the focus of class action suits by veterans. This chapter takes up the role of these diagnoses in the criminal justice system and in military disciplinary proceedings and how PTSD emerged as a site of psychiatric reforms. The chapter draws on my field interviews with staff and patients at a state psychiatric hospital—an important site of border conflict between the prisons and mental health systems—and shows how the PTSD category operates for staff in managing their conflicting roles as both therapists and prison guards. I also draw on my interviews with military clinicians and introduce historical cases to illustrate some of the bitter controversies in the past that continue to resurface in war zones. Distinctions between the war neuroses and character disorders have been a conflict zone in the military since World War I, and clinicians have brought trauma into the picture during this same long history to elicit greater sympathy for those accused of crimes in both military and civilian contexts. The concept of *moral injury*, introduced in Chapter 1, is developed further here to revisit an old controversy over how to clinically frame the psychologically destructive effects of warfare.

Chapter 3, "Psychic Trauma and the Body," looks at how stress and trauma models approach the body as the location for signs and symptoms related to PTSD. Clinicians are expected to identify medical problems and physical complaints that may contribute to the mental disorder or to co-existing conditions. I show how defending PTSD and its precursor conditions has often depended on its capacity to mimic a recognized medical condition. Historical cases are presented to explain the pressures on clinicians to reference medical knowledge to secure their own legitimacy as well as that of their patients' complaints. This reliance on symptoms associated with assaults on the body extends into the concept of moral injury as a condition associated with warfare.

Chapter 4, "Distressing and Disabling Conditions," extends my case study into the contentious ground of disability claims and how the medico-legal terrain of PTSD has been pivotal to psychiatry's role in adjudicating these claims. Veterans face a far less hostile political climate for their disability claims than do other groups. But there is a great deal to be learned from the history of veterans' struggles and the role of psychiatric experts in adjudicating their post-war complaints. The liberalizing of criteria for PTSD in military disability cases has been heralded as a progressive advance by veterans' advocates. But this chapter shows how PTSD diagnostic and narrative strategies inadvertently silence veterans and narrow public discourse over social welfare, along with the morally charged distinctions between the honorable and the dishonorable, the valorized and the damned, that the early movement sought to dismantle.

Chapter 5, "Suffering Together: Group Responses to Trauma," focuses on social movements that have shaped PTSD stories and demands on psychiatry to respond to those movements. Contemporary ethical guidelines for mental health professionals require that clinicians attend to the cultural significance of symptoms. As critiques of the mental health field mounted in the late 20th century, professionals increasingly embraced the PTSD diagnosis and trauma treatments as a way of responding to charges of cultural bias in the mental health field. PTSD offered a way of assigning a diagnosis that seemed to be immune to these critiques. The chapter enlists critical psychoanalytic traditions in tracking the migration of the diagnosis in the global field of humanitarian psychiatry and as it emerges as a defensive reaction for practitioners carrying out relief work in conflict zones. I draw on critics working in crisis zones, some of whom are working to "decolonize trauma theory," with others arguing for the dismantling of trauma diagnoses altogether.

Finally, the "Conclusions" chapter returns to the questions guiding this project on the role of psychiatry in addressing mental suffering. The touchstone ideas that informed the critical psychiatry/anti-psychiatry movement of the 1960s and 1970s are brought into these conclusions—ideas that include recognizing that people can be both crazy and sane, both impaired and creative, and that the generativity of the human mind carries multiple potentialities. This critical analysis points beyond the clinical encounter in seeking ways of listening and responding to people in distress, and of creating reparative community practices. At the same time, there is something to be said for Freud's old adage that the purpose of psychoanalysis is to transform neurotic misery into everyday unhappiness. Suffering is part of the human condition. But so, too, are human efforts to intervene in that suffering.

# References

Agel, J. (1971). *The radical therapist: The radical therapist collective* (English language edition). New York, NY: Ballantine Books.

Alford, C. F. (2009). *The Holocaust is not traumatic; the Holocaust can be represented.* Paper Presented at the Political Science Association Annual Meeting, Toronto, Canada.

American Psychiatric Association. (1987). *Diagnostic and statistical manual of mental disorders: DSM-III-R* (3rd ed., Rev ed.). Washington, DC: Author.

American Psychiatric Association. (2013). *Diagnostic and statistical manual of mental disorders (DSM-5)*. Washington, DC: Author.

Benjamin, J. (1988). *The bonds of love: Psychoanalysis, feminism, and the problem of domination*. New York, NY: Pantheon Books.

Benjamin, J. (2018). *Beyond doer and done to* (1st ed.). New York, NY: Routledge.

Berlim, M., & Fleck, M. P. (2003). Notes on antipsychiatry. *European Archives of Psychiatry and Clinical Neuroscience, 252*(2), 61–67.

Berrios, G. E. (1999). Classifications in psychiatry: A conceptual history. *Australian & New Zealand Journal of Psychiatry, 33*(2), 145–160.

Bremner, J. D., & Marmar, C. R. (2002). *Trauma, memory, and dissociation*. Washington, DC: American Psychiatric Association Publishing.

Breslau, J. (2004). Introduction: Cultures of trauma: Anthropological views of post-traumatic stress disorder in international health. *Culture, Medicine and Psychiatry, 28*(2), 113–126. https://doi.org/10.1023/B:MEDI.0000034421.07612.c8

Brewin, C. R., Lanius, R. A., Novac, A., Schnyder, U., & Galea, S. (2009). Reformulating PTSD for DSM-V: Life after Criterion A. *Journal of Traumatic Stress, 22*(5), 366–373. https://doi.org/10.1002/jts.20443

Callard, F. (2014). Psychiatric diagnosis: The indispensability of ambivalence. *Journal of Medical Ethics, 40*(8), 526–530. https://doi.org/10.1136/medethics-2013-101763

Camp, N. M. (2015). *US Army psychiatry in the Vietnam War: New challenges in extended counterinsurgency warfare*. Washington, DC: Government Printing Office.

Caruth, C. (1991). Unclaimed experience: Trauma and the possibility of history. *Yale French Studies, Literature and the Ethical Question* (79), 181–192. Retrieved from JSTOR.

Caruth, C. (2014). *Listening to trauma: Conversations with leaders in the theory and treatment of catastrophic experience*. Baltimore, MD: John Hopkins University Press.

Cheney, A. M., Koenig, C. J., Miller, C. J., Zamora, K., Wright, P., Stanley, R., . . . Pyne, J. M. (2018). Veteran-centered barriers to VA mental healthcare services use. *BMC Health Services Research, 18*(1), 591–605. https://doi.org/10.1186/s12913-018-3346-9

Chesler, P. (1997). *Women and madness* (3rd ed.). New York, NY: Four Walls Eight Windows.

Cohen, C. I. (1993). The biomedicalization of psychiatry: A critical overview. *Community Mental Health Journal, 29*(6), 509–521. https://doi.org/10.1007/BF00754260

Collins, P. H. (2000). *Black feminist thought: Knowledge, consciousness, and the politics of empowerment* (2nd ed.). New York, NY: Routledge.

Cooper, A. M. (1990). The future of psychoanalysis: Challenges and opportunities. *The Psychoanalytic Quarterly, 59*(2), 177–196. https://doi.org/10.1080/21674086.1990.11927269

Cors, C., Lau, S., & Farmer, D. J. (2013). Fragmented warrior: Fragmented administration. *Administrative Theory & Praxis, 35*(3), 424–437. https://doi.org/10.2753/ATP1084-1806350305

Craps, S., Cheyette, B., Gibbs, A., Andermahr, S., & Allwork, L. (2015). Decolonizing trauma studies round-table discussion. *Humanities, 4*(4), 905–923. https://doi.org/10.3390/h4040905

Cushman, P. (2002). How psychology erodes personhood. *Journal of Theoretical and Philosophical Psychology, 22*(2), 103–113.

Cushman, P. (2012). Defenseless in the face of the status quo: Psychology without a critical humanities. *The Humanistic Psychologist, 40*(3), 262–269. Retrieved from www.researchgate.net/publication/254314237_Defenseless_in_the_Face_of_the_Status_Quo_Psychology_without_a_Critical_Humanities

Dobbs, D. (2009). The post-traumatic stress trap. *Scientific American, 300*(4), 64–69.

Eghigian, G. (2010). *From madness to mental health: Psychiatric disorder and its treatment in Western civilization.* New Brunswick, NJ: Rutgers University Press.

Felman, S. (1992). Education and crisis, or the vicissitudes of teaching. In D. Laub & S. Felman (Eds.), *Testimony: Crises of witnessing in literature, psychoanalysis and history* (pp. 21–76). New York, NY: Routledge.

Freud, S. (1899/1962). Screen memories. In J. Strachey (Ed.), *The standard edition of the complete psychological works of Sigmund Freud, volume III (1893–1899): Early psycho-analytic publications*: Vol. III (pp. 299–322). London, UK: The Hogarth Press.

Frueh, B. C., Grubaugh, A. L., Elhai, J. D., & Buckley, T. C. (2007). US Department of Veterans Affairs disability policies for posttraumatic stress disorder: Administrative trends and implications for treatment, rehabilitation, and research. *American Journal of Public Health, 97*(12), 2143–2145. https://doi.org/10.2105/AJPH.2007.115436

Frueh, B. C., Hamner, M. B., Cahill, S. P., Gold, P. B., & Hamlin, K. L. (2000). Apparent symptom overreporting in combat veterans evaluated for PTSD. *Clinical Psychology Review, 20*(7), 853–885. https://doi.org/10.1016/S0272-7358(99)00015-X

Ganaway, G. K. (1989). Historical versus narrative truth: Clarifying the role of exogenous trauma in the etiology of MPD and its variants. *Dissociation: Progress in the Dissociative Disorders, 2*(4), 205–220.

Haaken, J. (1998). *Pillar of salt: Gender, memory, and the perils of looking back.* New Brunswick, NJ: Rutgers University Press.

Haaken, J. (2010). *Hard knocks: Domestic violence and the psychology of storytelling.* New York, NY: Routledge.

Haaken, J. (2014). *Mind zone: Therapists behind the front lines* [Documentary]. United States: Herzog & Company.

Haaken, J. (2016). Riding the waves of feminism: Psychoanalysis and women's liberation. *Psychoanalysis, Culture & Society, 21*(3), 223–231. https://doi.org/10.1057/pcs.2016.5

hooks, b. (1992). *Black looks: Race and representation*. Boston, MA: South End Press.

Isaacs, A. R. (2000). *Vietnam shadows: The war, its ghosts, and its legacy*. Baltimore, MD: Johns Hopkins University Press.

Kintsch, W., & Greene, E. (1978). The role of culture-specific schemata in the comprehension and recall of stories. *Discourse Processes*, *1*(1), 1–13. https://doi.org/10.1080/01638537809544425

Kleinman, A. (2012). Rebalancing academic psychiatry: Why it needs to happen—and soon. *The British Journal of Psychiatry*, *201*(6), 421–422. https://doi.org/10.1192/bjp.bp.112.118695

Kriss, S. (2013, October 18). *Book of lamentations*. Retrieved January 7, 2019, from The New Inquiry website: https://thenewinquiry.com/book-of-lamentations/

Laub, D. (2009). On Holocaust testimony and its "reception" within its own frame, as a process in its own right: A response to "Between History and Psychoanalysis" by Thomas Trezise. *History and Memory*, *21*(1), 127–150. https://doi.org/10.2979/HIS.2009.21.1.127

Levin, A. P., Kleinman, S. B., & Adler, J. S. (2014). DSM-5 and posttraumatic stress disorder. *Journal of the American Academy of Psychiatry and the Law Online*, *42*(2), 146–158.

Levy, M. I. (1995, November). Stressing the point: When are post traumatic stress claims legitimate . . . and when are they not? *For the Defense*. Retrieved from www.experts.com/Articles/Post-Traumatic-Stress-Disorder-Claim-By-Mark-Levy

Lewis-Fernández, R., & Kleinman, A. (1995). Cultural psychiatry: Theoretical, clinical, and research issues. *Psychiatric Clinics of North America*, *18*(3), 433–448.

Macpherson, M. (1981, March 15). Pulling the rug from under Vietnam Vets again. *Washington Post*. Retrieved from www.washingtonpost.com/archive/opinions/1981/03/15/pulling-the-rug-from-under-vietnam-vets-again/f06bbe51-063c-4886-8426-9b881e1f3a25/

McHugh, P. R., & Treisman, G. (2007). PTSD: A problematic diagnostic category. *Journal of Anxiety Disorders*, *21*(2), 211–222. https://doi.org/10.1016/j.janxdis.2006.09.003

McNally, R. J., & Frueh, B. C. (2013). Why are Iraq and Afghanistan War veterans seeking PTSD disability compensation at unprecedented rates? *Journal of Anxiety Disorders*, *27*(5), 520–526. https://doi.org/10.1016/j.janxdis.2013.07.002

Mezzich, J. E., Kirmayer, L. J., Kleinman, A., Fabrega, H., Parron, D. L., Good, B. J., . . . Manson, S. M. (1999). The place of culture in DSM-IV. *Journal of Nervous and Mental Disease*, *187*(8), 457–464.

Miller, A. (2006). *The body never lies: The lingering effects of hurtful parenting* (Reprint edition and A. Jenkins, Trans.). New York, NY: W. W. Norton & Company.

Nash, W. P., & Litz, B. T. (2013). Moral injury: A mechanism for war-related psychological trauma in military family members. *Clinical Child and Family Psychology Review*, *16*(4), 365–375.

Nasser, M. (1995). The rise and fall of anti-psychiatry. *The Psychiatrist*, *19*(12), 743–746. https://doi.org/10.1192/pb.19.12.743

Noble, R. C. (1993). Physicians and the pharmaceutical industry: An alliance with unhealthy aspects. *Perspectives in Biology and Medicine*, *36*(3), 376–394. https://doi.org/10.1353/pbm.1993.0010

Orsillo, S. M., Weathers, F. W., Litz, B. T., Steinberg, H. R., Huska, J. A., & Keane, T. M. (1996). Current and lifetime psychiatric disorders among veterans with war zone-related posttraumatic stress disorder. *Journal of Nervous and Mental Disease*, *184*(5), 307–313.

Parker, I. (2013). *The crisis in modern social psychology (psychology revivals) and how to end it* (1st ed.). https://doi.org/10.4324/9781315888569

Parker, I. (Ed.). (2015). *Handbook of critical psychology*. London, UK: Routledge.

Power, M. (2015). *Madness cracked* (1st ed.). London, UK: Oxford University Press.

Probst, B. (2014). The life and death of Axis IV: Caught in the quest for a theory of mental disorder. *Research on Social Work Practice*, *24*(1), 123–131.

Proctor, H. (2018, June 19). *Mad world: Radical psychiatry and 1968* [Blog]. Retrieved January 13, 2019, from Versobooks.com website: www.versobooks.com/blogs/3888-mad-world-radical-psychiatry-and-1968

Richardson, D. J., Sareen, J., Stein, M. B., & Ovuga, E. (2012). Psychiatric management of military-related PTSD: Focus on psychopharmacology. In *Post traumatic stress disorders in a global context* (pp. 51–70). London, UK: IntechOpen.

Ross, C. A. (1989). *Multiple personality disorder: Diagnosis, clinical features, and treatment*. Hoboken, NJ: Wiley-Interscience.

Scott, W. J. (1990). PTSD in DSM-III: A case in the politics of diagnosis and disease. *Social Problems*, *37*(3), 294–310.

Sedgwick, P. (1982). *Psycho politics: Laing, Foucault, Goffman, Szasz, and the future of mass psychiatry*. New York, NY: Harper & Row.

Shaw, R. (2007). Memory frictions: Localizing the Truth and Reconciliation Commission in Sierra Leone. *International Journal of Transitional Justice*, *1*(2), 183–207. https://doi.org/10.1093/ijtj/ijm008

Shaw, R. (2012). Displacing violence: Making Pentecostal memory in postwar Sierra Leone. *Cultural Anthropology*, *22*(1), 66–93.

Shay, J. (1994). *Achilles in Vietnam: Combat trauma and the undoing of character*. New York, NY: Simon and Schuster.

Shoeb, M., Weinstein, H., & Mollica, R. (2007). The Harvard trauma questionnaire: Adapting a cross-cultural instrument for measuring torture, trauma and posttraumatic stress disorder in Iraqi refugees. *International Journal of Social Psychiatry*, *53*(5), 447–463. https://doi.org/10.1177/0020764007078362

Stein, D. J., Phillips, K. A., Bolton, D., Fulford, K. W. M., Sadler, J. Z., & Kendler, K. S. (2010). What is a mental/psychiatric disorder? From DSM-IV to DSM-V. *Psychological Medicine*, *40*(11), 1759–1765.

Summerfield, D. (2001). The invention of post-traumatic stress disorder and the social usefulness of a psychiatric category. *BMJ: British Medical Journal*, *322*(7278), 95–98.

Ulman, R. B., & Brothers, D. (1988). *The shattered self: A psychoanalytic study of trauma*. Hillsdale, NJ: The Analytic Press.

van der Kolk, B. (2015). *The body keeps the score: Brain, mind, and body in the healing of trauma* (Reprint edition). New York, NY: Penguin Books.

Visser, I. (2015). Decolonizing trauma theory: Retrospect and prospects. *Humanities*, *4*(2), 250–265. https://doi.org/10.3390/h4020250

Watson, J. B. (1925). *Behaviorism*. New York, NY: People's Institute Publishing Company, Incorporated.

Wilson, M. (1993). DSM-III and the transformation of American psychiatry: A history. *American Journal of Psychiatry*, *150*(3), 399–410. https://doi.org/10.1176/ajp.150.3.399

Woollard, R. F. (1993). Addressing the pharmaceutical industry's influence on professional behaviour. *CMAJ: Canadian Medical Association Journal*, *149*(4), 403–404.

Young, A. (1997). *The harmony of illusions: Inventing post-traumatic stress disorder*. Princeton, NJ: Princeton University Press.

# Chapter 1

# Listening to Distressing Stories

How people integrate a terrible experience into their sense of self is a complex process. My own mother taught me as a young girl that it is better to be killed if you are raped. In her Christian worldview, it was better to die in purity than to live in sexual defilement. The women's movement of the 1970s organized to resist both rape and the stigma of rape—the idea that survivors were morally contaminated or "damaged goods." Yet filing charges against perpetrators through the courts often requires establishing damages or personal injury—a legal process that makes it difficult to prosecute an injustice without establishing that one has been psychologically impaired by the experience.

As a feminist and psychoanalytic clinician, I listen for these cultural echoes in how women talk about experiences of sexual assault. I recall a woman who came to see me years ago with a fairly common concern of women in their 30s. She wanted to get pregnant and have a child but was struggling with a reluctant and emotionally distant boyfriend. He seemed to have commitment issues. He had recently ushered her through a tour of the house he had purchased without her having seen the place. Additional signs pointed to poor prospects with this man: He was content with their weekly rituals of take-out dinners followed by tepid sex; he had no interest in having a child (although vaguely open to the possibility down the road); and an old girlfriend served as his general life advisor. Over the first six months of therapy, we explored her history of intimate relationships and what she experienced as her own disturbing lack of sexual desire, in palpable contrast to her growing longing for a baby. In one session, my patient described being a victim of rape several years prior. She had been working as a stripper at a local club and a customer followed her home. The man had crawled through her bathroom window, ripped off her skirt and raped her on the floor, then fled through the front door. She called 911 and the police arrived and took her report. She had no memory of the rapist's face, only recollections of the sickening smell of beer and the weight of his sweaty body on her frame and his penis jamming inside her. A police report was filed but my patient chose not to pursue the investigation.

As she described the events of that night, her account of the rape was bound up in her experience of working at the club. She had played over and over in her mind the sequence of events. As a pole dancer, there were rules for touching, and she did exercise control over customers. But there was always this uneasiness she felt driving home, wondering if something like this might happen. Shortly after the rape, she quit her job at the club and moved in with her parents, neither of whom knew she worked as a dancer. As we spoke about the rape, I was aware of her searching my face and looking for signs of disapproval. Would I place her in the same line-up of morally suspect victims to which the police seemed so ready to assign her in their questioning? Would I share the imagined reproaches of her parents? This rape did have a profound and lasting effect on my patient. Her suffering was heightened, however, by the disdainful attitude of the police and her aching aloneness at the time. In subtle ways, she had structured her daily activity to minimize situations that might remind her of the hideous residue of this man. Over the course of her therapy, the rape became part of her larger life-narrative.

PTSD treatments center on emotionally processing a memory—the Criterion A of the diagnosis thought to be the cause of the disorder. The question of whether my patient met the criteria for PTSD was not at issue in her therapy since her initial diagnosis of depression—dysthymic disorder—still described her symptoms. And she had not applied for victims' benefits through the state—a program that covers counseling and can require establishing a diagnosis of PTSD. A paradox of PTSD treatment, however, revolves around its tendency to reproduce a dynamic where the abuser remains at the center of the stage. Bessel van der Kolk (2015), for example, cautions that

> if a person does not remember, he is likely to act out: he reproduces it not as a memory but as an action; he repeats it, without knowing, of course, that he is repeating, and in the end, we understand that this is his way of remembering.
>
> (p. 183)

In this chapter, I show how the process of acting out—of unconsciously converting a conflict into modes of containing the conflict—applies as much to the clinician as it does to the patient.

All diagnoses carry the subjective judgments of the clinicians that assign them. They are shaped by *countertransference* reactions—responses to the patient based on associations with psychologically meaningful experiences in the therapist's own past. Just as the patient engages in transference reactions, so too does the therapist. But these judgments are mediated both by the professional culture that guides clinical thinking as well as through the dynamics of the therapist's personal history. In addition, as psychoanalyst Lynne Layton (2015) explains, clinical interpretations include unconscious identifications with the dominant culture and its ruling ideologies. One of those ideologies centers on over-investment in the power of the "talking cure" itself—the belief that emotional suffering is largely an individual problem requiring individual interventions. For clinicians working in institutional settings, whether state hospitals, the courts, schools, Veterans Administration, or the active military, the constraints on their own therapeutic powers and the range of individual choices available to their clients are palpably present. My interest has been to understand how clinicians in these settings use the PTSD diagnosis to manage those constraints.

## Clinical Storytelling

The DSM-5 (American Psychiatric Association, 2013) comments in its intro-duction that "we have come to recognize that the boundaries between disorders are more porous than originally perceived" (p. 6). The job of the clinician is to discern a picture within those porous boundaries. And although the diagnoses are partly based on statistical analysis of aggregate data, the practitioner sees one person at a time and hears one story at a time. In using the manual as a guide, practitioners must turn from the distressed person before them to the 950-page manual on the shelf and leaf through the hundreds of options avail-able for classification. For clinicians seeking to determine if the symptoms map onto the PTSD criteria, the ideal prototype is the person who presents with a story of a life-threatening recent event and reports how this event continues to preoccupy the person and interfere with functioning. As Richard McNally (2009) concludes in distilling the clinical essence of PTSD, the memory of the traumatic event is the "heart of the diagnosis" (p. 599).

In some institutional settings, PTSD signifies more of an attitude toward a patient than a diagnostic procedure. Most patients at the state hospital where I carried out interviews have histories of significant trauma, much of which is documented in charts filled with heartbreaking stories. But the daily real-ity is that the patients are prisoners confined to this institution because they have committed serious crimes. Conflict over their own dual roles as therapists and prison guards repeatedly arose in the course of making *Guilty Except for Insanity* (Haaken, 2013), a film about patients entering the Oregon State Hos-pital (OSH) through the insanity defense. In one scene in the film, staff are demonstrating how to administer five-point restraints in a way that conforms to legal and ethical standards. A high rate of using physical restraints on patients is an indicator of a poorly run psychiatric hospital. Staff at OSH took consid-erable pride in keeping rates of restraints low, even though staff defended the use of the practice with violent patients. In the film scene, four staff members surrounded the gurney to demonstrate how the restraints work. In the course of the scene, one of the nurses commented that "often patients come into the hospital with PTSD issues so you want to be respectful of their boundaries and the potential for triggering past trauma in holding them down. It can feel like an assault." She was part of a group at the hospital pushing for more trauma-based care—an approach that acknowledges how the institution and treatments administered can be traumatic for some patients.

In this demonstration of restraints, PTSD was invoked as a reminder that patients bring into the hospital histories not of their own making. This diagnostic lens provided a humanizing view of the resistive patient. Although admitted under the insanity plea, these patients were also viewed as victims of a mental illness. The evaluation process centers on determining whether the person is able to conform their behavior to the requirements of the law and whether a "mental disease or defect" impairs this capacity. By reminding co-workers that "this person may have PTSD issues," the staff member introduces a caveat. Restraints are acknowledged as potentially traumatizing. At the same time, the conflict over the harmful effects of restraints is externalized. The trauma is represented as an effect of the patient's past rather than as embedded in institutional practices. Further, invoking PTSD introduces a form of institutional splitting—avoidance of anxiety by keeping separate the two elements of a conflict, in this case the trauma produced through the restraints and the trauma that patients bring through their histories. The conflict associated with restraints is managed through separating patients into those vulnerable by way of their PTSD histories and those who are not vulnerable and thus evoke less concern.

Much like staff at the OSH, clinicians in the Veterans Affairs system are located at a site where they face conflicting pressures to both recognize the effects of warfare and bring these effects under control. Clinicians I interviewed in the course of my field work were keenly aware of their roles in managing a growing mental health crisis related to over a decade of ongoing and open-ended warfare. Therapists were under pressure to treat and prevent PTSD and other mental health disorders, while also maintaining the fighting forces (J. Sardo, personal communication, June 8, 2011; Russell, Schaubel, & Figley, 2018). Furthermore, the US Department of Defense and the VA system have emerged as primary sites for destigmatizing mental health problems, particularly through campaigns focused on recognizing symptoms of PTSD.

## Diagnostic Disputes

This book situates PTSD in the context of a crisis in psychiatry over its responsibility to intervene in socially produced suffering. Although the mental health field encompasses a wide range of disciplines and applied practices, the American Psychiatry Association, as author of the DSM, holds the leading role in developing a taxonomy of mental disorders. The anti-psychiatry movement of the 1960s and 1970s, along with the feminist and anti-war movements, took aim at psychiatry for its failure to address societal factors in the development of clinical syndromes and its collusion in the very problems that the profession claims to alleviate. In advancing this critique, British psychiatrist David Cooper (2001), an early leader in the anti-psychiatry movement, describes the treatment of people hospitalized "with what is called a 'schizophrenic breakdown'" and how psychiatry as a profession is "co-operating in the systematic invalidation of a wide category of persons" (p. xi). This early critique centered on the position of psychiatric hospitals in the institutional control over behaviors cast as deviant. But as the PTSD diagnosis gained official recognition, it became symptomatic of a wider crisis in psychiatry over its role in the social management of suffering. Part of this crisis centered on challenges to culturally hegemonic notions of normalcy, and of the role of psychiatry in codifying differences between variations along a continuum of normalcy and behaviors that cross some threshold into mental pathology.

The PTSD movement generated adherents in the late 20th century through its insistence that normal people can appear quite mentally disturbed when confronted with extreme situations (Herman, 1992; Litz et al., 2009). The question of what constitutes "normal experience" has generated considerable ongoing debate, however, in the wake of PTSD's entry into the DSM (Brewin, Lanius, Novac, Schnyder, & Galea, 2009; Malik & Beutler, 2002). The diagnosis presupposed a circumscribed event that departed from some idyllic conception of normal life. The initial model was also based on exposure to events bound in time and place. Critics pointed out the class and race premises of the diagnoses and posed further questions: Is living in a violent household a normal experience? What about homeless people or those living under police-state conditions in cities or asylum seekers along the US/Mexico border? Who defines departures from normalcy? And what about military forms of PTSD where soldiers are serving multiple deployments over many years? Even in the PTSD prototypes of war and rape, the diagnosis tended to focus on a dramatic story based on a single event.

PTSD stands alone in the DSM as a disorder defined by its cause. It developed as part of a campaign initiated by anti-war clinicians and veterans' groups to address the long-term consequences of warfare. Yet the question of etiology—how to identify the *cause* of a disorder—remains one of the more elusive controversies in the field of psychiatry (Brewin, Andrews, & Valentine, 2000; Brunner, 2000; Davidson & Foa, 1993; Hurst, 1917; Kinzie & Goetz, 1996). Although uncertainties over causality underlie the entire system of psychiatric classification, PTSD became a lightning rod in the late 20th and early 21st centuries for this seemingly intransigent problem. Humans gather up a vast array of formative experiences over time that shape the clinical picture. Indeed, the push in the PTSD field to develop procedures for identifying Criterion A—the "index trauma"—proceeded out of step with the larger trend in psychiatry toward recognizing multiple etiological factors. Research on genetics points to a complex web of determinants that contribute to mental disorders, and to the hundreds of genes that may play a role. The genome project fell short of expectations in the 1990s in clarifying these muddy etiological waters (Koenen, 2007; Yehuda, 2006). As DSM Work Group members

Robert Spitzer and Michael First (2005) confess in summarizing the work of the fourth edition of the manual:

> Little progress has been made toward understanding the pathophysiological processes and etiology of mental disorders. If anything, the research has shown the situation is even more complex than initially imagined, and we believe not enough is known to structure the classification of psychiatric disorders according to etiology.
>
> (p. 1898)

This proclamation attests to the limits of psychiatry's claims of direct parallels between mental and physical illness as well. There are no consistent biological markers or tests for most mental disorders (Kleinman, 2012; Yehuda, 2006). The disorders are based on *groupings* of behavioral indicators, many of which would not be considered pathological in a different cultural or historical context (Good, Good, Hyde, & Pinto, 2008; Kleinman, 2011). In a sense, all mental disorders are *syndromes*—a term that admits to limited knowledge concerning underlying etiology of observed signs and symptoms. Even the term *disorder*, which replaced the less clinical term *reactions* in the first versions of the DSM manual, signifies the murky linguistic terrain of psychiatry. Disorders are not diseases in the medical sense, but they do point to deviations from normalcy. Since mental health professionals differ widely in the theories of etiology they bring to the diagnostic process, the DSM committee sought scientific consensus on the basis of statistical correlations—groups of symptoms that seem to co-occur across a broad range of clinical cases.

The psychiatric search for predictable categories confronts a series of shifting borders at the descriptive level as well. As Frueh and colleagues (2000) frame the diagnostic dilemma, "there is (a) a profound lack of symptom discrimination, and (b) a puzzling inconsistency in the obtained psychometric profiles and general clinical presentation (e.g., outpatient status) of many combat veterans evaluated for PTSD" (p. 856). The depressed person is often anxious, and the anxious person may become depressed. Drugs developed for one condition, such as psychosis, are often later promoted to treat other conditions, such as eating disorders. This cross-category use of medications is partly a function of marketing by drug companies. But it also is an effect of the nature of psychiatric conditions. They are fluid registers of mental disturbance based on a wide and fluctuating array of historical, cultural, psychological, and biological factors.

David Dobbs (2009) points out that the uniqueness of the PTSD diagnosis "also makes it uniquely problematic, for the tie is really to the memory of an event" (p. 66). Further, Dobbs explains how clinical research on PTSD has not generally incorporated findings in the larger field of memory studies—findings emphasizing the constructed nature of recollections (Loftus & Ketcham, 1996; Patihis, Ho, Tingen, Lilienfeld, & Loftus, 2014). When PTSD gained momentum during the 1980s, the mental health field was entering a period of struggle over establishing the veracity of traumatic memories. Hypnosis and guided imagery, as well as conventional exploratory techniques, were enlisted to uncover memories of early childhood trauma. But human memory is recognized today as far more complex than was understood in the 1980s, when a more realist version of representations of the past prevailed in the mental health field. The common assumption at the time was that traumatic memories could be repressed but preserved on an unconscious level—in dissociated states—that retain a fidelity to the original event.

Military-related PTSD stories are no less subject to the imaginative and reconstructive processes of memory than are other stories. Although veterans are as apt as any group to produce faulty memories of their experiences, the military PTSD literature subsumes such reports under "malingering," "lying," and "factitious PTSD" (McNally & Frueh, 2013; Newman & Schum, 1983). These morally charged terms reflect the suspicions and judgments often surrounding PTSD cases and institutional commitment to ferreting out true cases from their simulated look-alikes.

Some version of this fortifying of the PTSD boundaries has been replayed with each wave of revisions in the DSM. Whereas Criterion A in DSM-IV allowed for situations where a person experiences or witnesses an event outside of normal experience, DSM-5 Criterion A requires that the person experience a *life-threatening* event or major threat to physical integrity—or that the person had directly observed or experienced such a threat to a close person, such as a family member (Levin, Kleinman, & Adler, 2014). Rather than departure from normalcy, the traumatic stressor in DSM-5 is described in the stricter terms of its potential lethality.

This reworking of Criterion A failed to open a clear passage, however, for reining in the diagnosis. Like the obsessives' efforts to control areas of life that elude their habitual coping strategies, the DSM committee was caught in a vicious cycle. One dynamic of this cycle centered on the problem of how to uncouple trauma as it was used to classify events from trauma as a clinical response (Ozner & Weiss, 2004). If the magnitude of the threat failed to explain the symptomatology, researchers reasoned that differential PTSD rates must be based on preexisting factors. From World War I through the Vietnam War, military psychiatrists have argued that symptoms do not persist in mentally stable people. This was the premise most directly challenged by the PTSD movement, which argued that normal people can seem very crazy under crazy conditions. Yet the advocacy side of the PTSD movement had never directly dealt with the finding that most people in fact do not develop the clinical syndrome.

## The Suffering of Soldiers

As far back as the late 19th century, clinicians have reported cases where normal people exhibit psychiatric symptoms in response to extreme duress—a history taken up in later chapters of this book. But prior to the PTSD movement, the general assumption in the mental health field was that most people return to baseline functioning within weeks or months following a major stressful event. Military research on sustained exposure to extreme stressors, such as combat, acknowledges that breakdowns in functioning can be severe and potentially disabling. In a paper ominously titled "The Darker Side of Military Mental Healthcare," Russell et al. (2018) describe a series of lessons learned and subsequently repressed by the military concerning the long-term psychiatric impacts of warfare. In describing the defenses involved in this pattern of institutional repression, the authors point to how the use of the VA allows the Department of Defense to distance itself from the problem. "The present-day policy disavows responsibility or provision of mental health treatment and rehabilitation of veterans in the criminal justice system and foists the responsibility on the VA and private sector" (p. 47). Military research from World War I through the Vietnam War invested in screening procedures to separate those vulnerable to breakdowns from those normal men who were thought to be equipped to withstand the rigors of warfare (Nash & Litz, 2013).

Early PTSD advocates argued that normal people could develop symptoms years or even decades after their exposure to a major stressor. Anti-war activists lobbied a DSM sub-committee for inclusion of post-Vietnam syndrome, a condition characterized by an inability to mourn and by feelings of guilt, rage, and betrayal. Psychiatrist and anti-war activist Chaim Shatan (1972) offered a profile: "The post-Vietnam syndrome confronts us with the unconsummated grief of soldiers' 'impacted grief' in which an encapsulated, never-ending past deprives the present of meaning" (p. 35). More than a diagnosis of individual psychopathology, this description was an indictment of a society blinded by idealized images of the American military and prone to repressing the disturbing and lasting consequences of warfare. As medical anthropologist Kenneth MacLeish (2018) observes, however, veterans' displays of mental anguish have carried their own demand characteristics, reassuring the public that "soldiers' pain is a sign of their humanity" (p. 140). Societal anxieties over returning service members animate some of these public demands, including appeals on websites offering mental health services for morally injured veterans.

The pressures on clinicians to return troubled veterans to normalcy shape thresholds for hearing and making sense of the material at hand. One scene of tension centers on what to call the conditions of disturbed soldiers in war zones. The term *traumatic war neurosis* was commonly used in military psychiatry during the latter part of World War I and up through World War II, although the military avoids diagnosing soldiers until they are evacuated from combat zones. In both the UK and the US military, *shell shock* was abandoned as a term because it was too bound to physical impacts and too narrow in the conditions it encompassed. Physicians increasingly diagnosed cases of shell shock far from the front and many noted the psychological complexity of reactions to warfare (Southard, 1919)—a lesson taken into World War II military psychiatry (Gilbert, 1983; Kardiner, 1941). Unlike shell shock, the concept of a war neurosis conceded that a range of situations in the theater of war could produce a psychiatric illness. The term *neuro-psychiatric* disorders gained favor during World War II as military doctors sought to dispel suspicions surrounding mental breakdowns through a closer affinity with neurology, a less controversial field of medicine than psychiatry.

The jettisoning of the term war neurosis in the DSM was part of a larger shift away from the psychodynamic theory of *neurosis*, a term replaced in DSM-III by *anxiety-based disorder* (and reclassified again in DSM-5 under a separate category of trauma and stress conditions). Yet the concept of neurosis still holds validity in many clinical fields and everyday vernacular. Since a neurosis is conceptualized as a pattern of abnormal behavior organized around anxiety and unconscious defenses, the construct itself ran counter to behavioral approaches to psychiatry. Behaviorists focus on discrete observable signs—maladaptive responses to identifiable stimuli—and reject models that look for underlying (unconscious) dynamics. Psychoanalysts attempt to understand the symbolic significance of a neurotic symptom. In hearing a patient tell a story about fear of leaving the house (agoraphobia), for example, the analyst might explore how this fear both signals and serves to repress less consciously accessible concerns, such as conflicts concerning independence. Behaviorists, on the other hand, focus on the more immediate set of stimuli or contingencies that produce this irrational fear. Both psychoanalytic and behavioral approaches accept that the phobia serves some initial adaptive function while becoming more limiting as the person relies too heavily on this mode of coping. Psychoanalysts would view the problem within the framework of a dynamic model of mind rather than as a discrete behavior that can be isolated from the mind as a system. In heated contestations over definitions of mental disorders, the DSM committee reasoned that clinicians of differing theoretical perspectives could agree that PTSD symptoms are reactions to an event or events that extend beyond a normal period of time. The traumatic event, the "index trauma," assumed an increasingly important role in diagnostic decision-making as the place in the road where everyone meets.

PTSD garnered support among veterans in part because it conveys a certain respect for warriors whose troubles are in the area of holding too tightly and for too long to their psychological armor as fighters. But the seeming universality of the condition had the effect of isolating clinical reactions from the larger military milieu. PTSD was both a story about the troubles that service members brought home with them and a condition thought to afflict all of humanity.

## Infantry Stories

Confusion over how to represent the experiences of veterans of differing military conflicts permeates the visual space as one enters the hallways where VA therapeutic and transition services are provided—the Operation Iraqi

Freedom/Operation Enduring Freedom (OIF/OEF) office. On entering, the visitor is greeted with the usual paraphernalia scattered about veterans' clinics: old issues of *Stars and Stripes*, bulletin boards with thumbtacked photos of young soldiers sitting erect on MRAP tanks (mine-resistant ambush protected) or goofing around with buddies in T-shirts, and educational posters with wind-swept American flags.

The OIF/OEF staff impressed me from the start. Stepping into the office one Monday morning to talk with staff about my documentary project, I was greeted by John King, a volunteer Army veteran. As I extended a hand in greeting, King responded without hesitation, reaching out with a hand scarred by third-degree burns and missing several fingers. He also flashed a boyish grin. In addition to staffing the reception desk, King spoke frequently at Yellow Ribbon gatherings for returning veterans and their families, laying out some of the challenges in disengaging psychologically from war. King was the best salesperson I had met in promoting VA services, particularly one-on-one counseling, which he claimed had saved his life. Actually, it was Darla Darville, a social worker with a broad and winsome smile and senior to the younger staff in the OIF/OEF office, who King specifically credited with pulling him back from the edge. He joked that they had forgotten to wear their Darla fan T-shirts that day—an unabashed expression of the warm regard for this woman known for her skills in calming down the most agitated of veterans. Both agreed to be part of the film and to publicly share their stories.

King wanted to become a social worker like Darville but faced high hurdles in getting there. Although he was a skilled public speaker, and clearly very smart, stepping into a college classroom filled him with waves of acute nausea. He tells the story of throwing up on his first day of class, his body violently refusing the entire educational experience. He explained that the real psychological issue for him was control. In the classroom, someone else—the instructor—was in charge. Although many students bring childhood conflicts into their battles with their teachers, King's history as an infantryman left him with a gut-level queasiness about submitting to authority. A sergeant in an infantry unit during the Iraq surge of 2006, King prided himself on being a strong leader. In the course of our interviews, he told the story several times of how he almost died during an attack on the Bradley tank carrying his unit into Baghdad. He explained how his squad unit was called to bring batteries to a tanker, arriving to find the gunner asleep with a brand-new second lieutenant from West Point in charge, the "so-called cream of the crop" King added sarcastically.

Softening in tone, he describes the ominous scene as his tank rolled up to find the entire unit taking a nap in a combat zone. He explains how difficult it is to maintain your edge after so many months of fighting, as well as the impassive resignation to death that becomes part of the combat syndrome:

> This guy goes to sleep, of course, Joe on the gun. Joe falls asleep too because there's not another guy awake with him up there. He shouldn't be

sleeping out in the combat zone anyways. Who could, right? But there's that disassociation again. You're totally, you're just, *whatever* you know? If they're going to get me, they're going to get me. Whatever. Hopefully it's quick, you know.

King explains how battle fatigue—a term that gained currency during the madness of trench warfare during World War I—goes beyond mere exhaustion. It merges with the wish to die that is itself a part of the psychology of war. Many psychological conditions involve a preoccupation with death, as Freud theorized in *Beyond the Pleasure Principle* (Caruth, 1991). But preoccupation with death holds a particular affinity with warfare, where soldiers often describe the wish to turn the lethal destructiveness and implements of war against the self (Lifton, 1985). During the four times we met for interviews, John often returned to the soldiers who died the day his tank was torched.

While badly injured and deeply scarred by the explosion, King exhibited what the military calls "resilience." Resilience training involves techniques for overcoming "catastrophizing"—the tendency common among depressives to over-generalize from small events, seeing ominous thunderstorms in every cloudy sky. In pre-deployment trainings, the focus on positive thinking makes sense as a form of cognitive control over anxiety. Rather than focusing on the negatives, resilience trainers instruct, it is helpful to remind oneself of the positives: "I have survived this and have many reasons to expect good things to happen in the future. Let's list those reasons." Rather than posttraumatic stress, proponents of this model speak of "posttraumatic growth" (Tedeschi & McNally, 2011). But it can seem absurd—even insane—to apply the simplistic techniques of positive psychology to situations where service members are struggling to manage actual combat, as well as the less dramatic but nonetheless dark moments of deployment.

There is a more relational way of thinking about psychological resilience, however: the capacity to make use of human connections in the face of the destructiveness of warfare. The existentialist psychiatrist Victor Frankl (1976) described this dynamic in accounting for the capacity of many concentration camp victims to survive psychologically. As a doctor and Holocaust survivor who combined personal testimony and clinical observations, Frankl extended the study of war conditions to concentration camp survivors. He identified factors that help people preserve their psychological integrity in horrifyingly dehumanizing situations—insights carrying implications for reactions to warfare more broadly. Those in support roles are less apt to suffer psychological trauma, Frankl suggests, because they are able to hold on to knowledge of themselves as good people. Much of the resilience training rolled out as part of the combat stress control training emphasizes cognitive techniques for reinterpreting events. But service members often struggle with the more difficult question of how to hold onto a sense of themselves as moral agents in the context of mass destructiveness (Lifton, 1985; Shay, 2003).

John King implicitly understood this principle. His stories abruptly shifted from the depravities of combat to the deep caring among comrades that emerges from the same inferno. Beginning with the bitter story of a complacent officer and exhausted troops waiting for death to overtake them, he turns to heroic accounts of fellow soldiers pulling his burning body from the Bradley, even as the soldiers under his command perished in that same tank.

The devastating trauma of that day became the basis of King's psychological disability—his PTSD "index trauma"—as well as his physical disability. It was a riveting and heartbreaking story, and the emotions coursing through the account were not readily condensed into the checklists available for PTSD assessment. There was the medic who held him together emotionally and physically in applying pressure dressings. And there was the story of his mother and girlfriend who stayed at his bedside in the nightmarish scenes of the burn unit, and caring doctors and nurses who patched his scorched body back together. King prided himself on his steely will but held a deep sense of gratitude for those who carried him through the hallucinatory horrors of those traumatic months. But there were countless other precursors to the trauma as well—moments when he realized that he no longer cared about the little Iraqi kids that crowded around the American troops, hawking knock-off DVDs and asking for candy. He recalled wondering some days about the parents of these kids who seemed to have disappeared from the scene. He thought about the old women who walked by and their weary looks as American tanks rolled through their towns. And he remembered the point where he "no longer gave a shit," hating everyone and only caring about the survival of his Joes. Operation New Dawn had dimmed to a dark night of the soul.

Over the course of our interviews, King's ambivalence about the military also surfaced as a palpable motif in his PTSD narrative. He was a hard-ass, pushing his men—his "Joes"—and having little tolerance for "sallies"—Joes who could not hold up under the rigors of combat. The only cause worth fighting for was other Joes, the band of brothers, and "America, apple pie and all of that" was bullshit. King's psychology of combat training was simple and straightforward: You get them to do what you want them to do, right now, and any attention to feelings was a distraction from the main job, which increasingly became survival. He also knew that good leaders are caring and expect no more from their soldiers than they expect of themselves. This is part of the tension between non-commissioned officers (NCOs)—who are like the shop floor supervisors laboring side by side with workers—and the more remote control of commissioned officers trained in military academies and university ROTC programs.

The heavy weight of this psychic armor produces wear and tear over time, not readily perceived in the short run. The combat role requires a tough hide—the capacity to dissociate—which can be difficult to separate from the pathological dissociation associated with PTSD. Indeed, unraveling the "index trauma" from the everyday stresses of the infantryman requires careful clinical parsing, eluding even the most refined diagnostic tools. Even as the notion of an index trauma locates responsibility for the suffering in the externalities of war, this framing of the soldier's problems makes it difficult to address the web of psychological and social dynamics that set the stage for the Criterion A event and what the service member brings to that experience. In structuring the exploration of memory around a stable and readily located scene, the DSM-authorized PTSD narrative forecloses on this wider stage of determinants.

In the course of my field work on military bases, I became aware of my own reactions to members of the military. I had a certain resistance to the Soldier's Story and to the special privileges granted male veterans for their service. Since I taught in a big state university, many veterans enrolled in my classes, but I had kept some distance from them. I tended to view them as willing instruments of US military aggression. In making the documentary, this hostility gave way to affection and respect for many service members and to an awareness of my own ambivalence about those employed in the US Armed Forces. Yet I found that many veterans shared this same ambivalence. As themes emerged in discussion of the meaning of soldiers' experiences of war, it became apparent that the PTSD treatments authorized by the military and VA systems tend to "repress" many of these emotional and existential aspects of post-deployment reactions.

## Transference Dynamics and the Theater of War

A central aim of psychoanalytic therapies is to understand *transference* reactions—how important experiences and formative relationships in the past are revived and revisited in the present. Yet, therapeutic exploration of this complex terrain confronts a political problem that gave rise to the PTSD movement: Personal histories were routinely used to discredit claimants. The PTSD codification of the index trauma—Criterion A—signified an important challenge to this use of psychiatry. Yet, like so many other coping strategies, this exclusion rule proved to be costly over time as it was codified and integrated into the medico-forensic reasoning of the DSM. Some of the costs take the form of limits on how people are able to understand and come to terms with their own experiences.

There were never questions in the VA disability system about the basis of John King's conditions—both medical and psychiatric—nor of the role of combat in producing them. The clarity of his case may have permitted him a degree of ease in talking about how his childhood set the stage for his aspirations as a soldier as well as for certain psychological vulnerabilities. Describing himself as the product of a "hippie, leftist lesbian mother" and a "cowboy right-wing father," John shifts in the course of minutes between these places on social identification. There is a notable sweetness about him, a bearing that conveys the impression of someone who has been loved, perhaps even adored. But stories of his father tower above all else in childhood memory. "She tried her best to keep me away from toy guns and aggression when I was a little kid," John explains in describing his mother, "but I had this big looming tough guy mountain man for a father you know, that a young guy is just going to be attracted to." This mountain of a man was clearly the object of intense ambivalence—of bitter hatred but also of respect.

"I hate to get into daddy issues," John wryly comments, "but the military does do that." Pulling out a photo of himself as a young boy reaching for the hand of this erectly postured man, John offers a self-analysis of his attraction to the military. "I always wanted to try to get him to be proud of me, and one off-comment one day about the military and being a man, and you're a sally if you don't go into the military . . . set the tone for the rest of my life." Keenly attuned to hypocrisy, John added that his father did not himself join up. There was a competitive dynamic that ran through this story, a sense of pride in beating his dad at his own manliness game. John finished the story of his dad by saying that "hopefully I broke that cycle." There is an allusion here to the intergenerational transmission of emotional struggle, with sons taking up the lost causes of fathers.

John would frequently comment on the hypocrisies of men who love the military but hate actual service, powerful old men who eagerly offer up the young to fight their vainglorious battles. The military requires a lot, John notes, but it gives a lot back, particularly to young people who are at a time in life when they are seeking recognition from parental substitutes. "When you do good, you're taken care of. When you really push yourself, people notice. And it feels good. It feels real good." Repeating the point for emphasis, John then shifts to a more cynical tone. "The military has a knack for getting young folks into thinking the way they want them to think. Especially infantry. *Real* good at it."

The love side of military ambivalence goes beyond attachment to superiors, however. Military service can unify in progressive ways. The Army was the first American institution to desegregate. Military experience carries many service members beyond the racially and geographically bounded locales of childhood. Indeed, spending time on military bases can feel like a socialist version of America—places where there are no major disparities in income levels, where there is a level of racial integration in working, eating, and living that is unheard of elsewhere in the country, and where people have their basic needs met and share a common commitment to service. Further, many MOS (military occupational specialty) jobs involve skills for which there are few applications on the civilian side. Yet this comradeship is in the service of military missions. As the Soldiers' Creed dictates, "I stand ready to deploy, engage, and destroy the enemies of the United States of America in close combat."

Although women were not allowed to join the infantry during his time of service, John expresses admiration for the female soldiers who regularly go "outside the wire"—beyond the protection of forward operating bases. These female soldiers often go on patrol or occupy support roles where they take considerable risks. Yet everyone in the military admires the infantry, he states emphatically. "We're the tip of the spear. They call us the queen of battle." The vast support systems in place to keep infantry in the fight affirm the prestige of the fighters.

The concept of *identification*—central to psychoanalytic formulations of human development—may be usefully employed in explaining relational dynamics associated with the war neuroses. The warrior initially enters into a potent identification with the military unit and its cultural codes, forged through submission to superiors. Idealization of the commander—as the good father figure—operates as a means of containing conflict within the group. The shared belief in the righteousness of the mission—as represented by the commander—keeps at bay feelings of doubt, uncertainty, and fear. John describes this intoxicating sense of invulnerability, often accompanied by flickering recognition of the chaos on the periphery: "when they're getting ready to send these guys over to combat zones, you think you're unstoppable. . . . We were ready to go in there and kick ass. We could not wait."

Psychoanalysis emphasizes the central role of narcissism in human development and the importance of expanded capacities for attachments in developing healthy forms of narcissism and ego strength. Human development begins with what Freud termed "His majesty the baby," with the lessons of life slowly and steadily requiring that the baby relinquish its reign (Freud, 1914/1957). Freud also notes how many psychological problems involve some failure to relinquish the position of His Majesty. And Freud recognized as well the gendered character of many narcissistic conditions, and the image of the phallus within a masculine symbolic order organized around warding off states of vulnerability. Many masculine maladies involve difficulties in acknowledging feelings of helplessness, vulnerability, or dependency, all of which contribute to a projection of strength that conceals an underlying fragility.

The trauma stories of many former infantrymen like John King are inseparable from their conflicted relationships with the military itself. Yet this relational context is strikingly absent in the checklists and treatments produced by and for the military. And this context centers on a fight for recognition that transcends the battles with official enemies. The story opens with a fighter enlisting the group to flee feminine identifications—to not be cast as a "sally"—in forging a sense of masculine invincibility. As fighters confront resistance or violence at the hands of the enemy, a second phase of the syndrome sets in. The narcissistic state of invulnerability is shattered. John describes these prototypical moments when things start to collapse and rage and revenge become the fuel that keeps them going. "Well, when people start dying around you, especially when they're people you care about, you're not looking at the political side of the house anymore. You don't care. You hate them." Reflecting on that state of hatred, John shakes his head. "It's awful. It's awful."

Battlefield breakdowns, described over the history of warfare, often involve the unauthorized use of violence. Soldiers may turn their weapons away from designated enemies and toward their comrades, officers, civilians, or themselves. Prosecuting service members who engage in such violence often involves assessment of their mental states—and whether they have suffered a traumatic stressor or brain injury that impairs reality testing or their capacity to exercise military discipline and good judgment. What these dramatic cases illustrate—and as readily obscure—are the everyday expressions of acting out in the theater of war. Manic behavior can be a desperate flight from terrifying feelings of vulnerability. Battlefield bravado often has this character of a frenetic escape from a desperate state of helplessness. Stress control clinicians may be called in at this juncture to manage a situation where a firefight is followed by reckless behavior. The question of what happened in the firefight is typically addressed in a highly restrictive way, with questions about the wisdom of the leadership or the mission itself explicitly forbidden. In hearing about these briefings from both therapists and veterans, John's own hardline opposition to battlefield psychiatry began to make sense. Debriefings offer a kind of safety valve for powerful emotions—rage, terror, helplessness, sadness. But it is difficult to gauge the safety of those release valves. Combat Stress Control clinicians often described these interventions as "force multipliers"—ways of getting more out of military "assets." This mission focus means that thoughts and feelings contrary to the mission tend to get repressed—psychologically and politically—until post-deployment. On some level, even the most committed of soldiers know they are being managed.

For some soldiers, there can be a fourth phase—a depressive reaction that often involves withdrawal of emotional investment in the mission. Service members often self-diagnose their response to this moment of crisis, explaining how the only thing that comes to matter is the buddy on your left and the buddy on your right. "I was there for Joe, I was there for the guy next to me," John declares, echoing countless other service members. "I can't look at it as I was there to help the Iraqi people, the Afghani people. . . . Bullshit. That's not why we're there." John extends the category of "Joes," perhaps in recognition of the many women surrounding and supporting him. "I mean it's for Joe. For Joe, right? Guy next to you, the gal next to you."

This narrow field of intense attachments—what clinicians term *traumatic bonding*—is partly cultivated by the military and partly a natural response to extreme situations. As John notes with some sympathy, the psychic apparatus of combat unravels on the home front. "These guys came from absolute total brotherhood to nothing, to just being lost . . . they feel alone, they don't have that support channel to fall back on." With some impatience, he describes the state of extreme dependency cultivated by the military, the unacknowledged part of military culture concealed behind the *Army Strong* bravado trumpeted on recruitment videos. When they return home, "they don't have Sergeant

King to make sure their bills are paid, to take care, you know, they don't have that anymore."

## Moral Awakenings

The PTSD clinical literature tends to overlook the importance of depressive reactions in holding on to one's humanity. From a Kleinian psychoanalytic perspective, human moral development depends on integrating into mind what Melanie Klein describes as the depressive state—recognizing one's capacity for destructiveness, hate, and envy, including against loved objects (see Alford, 1989; Burack, 2002). For some soldiers, fighting provides the primary psychological defense against depressive withdrawal, even as it may be directed at unauthorized targets. Acts of torture, rape, or other forms of violent assault represent an attempt to externalize an internal threat—to place it somewhere else, far from the precarious internal world that is on the verge of collapse. For others, the relationship to buddies in the unit acquires a heightened intensity. Everything outside of this fiercely protective sphere is of no value.

A sub-genre of PTSD storytelling focuses on the *moral injuries* of war—the sense of having been deeply damaged through either observing or participating in military missions that violate one's personal ethics or moral values (Litz et al., 2009; Nash, 2006; Nash & Litz, 2013; Shay, 2014). The concept captures some of the remainder of PTSD as a condition reduced to psychophysiological reactions—a gathering up of the troubling currents that have always dogged the psychiatric classifiers. Jonathan Shay (2003, 2014), a psychiatrist and prominent PTSD scholar, echoes the stances of others in the field who accept the narrowing of the diagnosis but seek to recoup the early movement's ethos through this looser clinical category of moral injury. As the Shay Moral Injury Center (n.d.) states on their website, "post-traumatic stress disorder is fear-based. Moral injury is not." The site goes on to explain that "moral injury has no diagnosis or treatment protocols." The recent surge of enthusiasm among clinicians for this concept represents a form of revolt against psychiatric protocols and checklists.

In listening to John's story, I was aware of his repeated reference to his moral awakening to the costs of warfare—a different concept than moral injury. Moral injury is a metaphor, just as is moral awakening. But moral injury achieves its rhetorical effects through its association with external blows, much like shell shock. Moral awakening suggests a disturbing stirring of some kind, akin to insight, that carries a set of social or ethical obligations. Injury requires attentiveness to one's wounds and represents a demand for care. Awakening, much like the idiom of being "woke," implies an enlargement of capacities rather than diminished capacities, but it also carries more of a focus on other-directed reparative efforts.

Clinicians working with veterans frequently talk about racism as an effect of war, although this rarely appears on the PTSD profiles of index troubles.

Problems with anger, explosive rage, and encounters with police are on these lists, but the scenes themselves and their cast of characters are less apt to generate scrutiny. John describes what he terms a post-deployment syndrome where the veteran continues to track the enemy in the form of hate directed to racial minorities and "foreigners." He came to recognize this dynamic as both a legacy of the military, with its dehumanizing of groups targeted as enemies, and part of the hyper-vigilance associated with combat conditions.

Psychologist Lori Daniels, a therapist at the Portland Vet Center, describes a dynamic where combat veterans move from racist hostility toward the enemy, ranting about "gooks" or "ragheads," to connecting with the humanity of the enemy (personal communication, May 14, 2011). She describes states of anxiety alongside shared identification with the enemy as the "other"—and that this disturbing awareness is often part of the intrusive images and disturbing memories routinely ascribed to PTSD. Rather than moral injury, she interprets this state as a form of moral awakening. Developing capacities for experiencing guilt and grief are central to group therapy, Daniels explains, although she adds that not all combat veterans experience such states. From her perspective, PTSD symptoms represent a stirring of feelings repressed behind the emotional deadness and depersonalization cultivated in warfare. The PTSD story, for Daniels, centers not simply on the experience of being damaged but on coming to terms with one's own capacity for destructiveness.

## Women's War Stories

The US military began to systematically enforce a new wave of tough policies around sexual assault in the early years of the 2000s. With women veterans suffering rates of PTSD similar to those of their male counterparts but encountering less combat (Street, Vogt, & Dutra, 2009), the problem of sexual harassment and assault took center stage as a leading cause of female war-related disabilities—an Agent Orange in the symbolic terrain of warfare. Although many researchers and clinicians point out that military sexual trauma (MST) is not just a women's issue, gender dynamics are certainly at the center of the story. MST is most often framed as a correlative of PTSD (Kimerling, Gima, Smith, Street, & Frayne, 2007; Street & Stafford, 2009). Within the military context, sexual trauma has been shown to pose at least as great a risk for PTSD as combat exposure (Kimerling et al., 2007). The VA introduced MST as a category associated with PTSD, along with Department of Defense mandated trainings and screenings. The public pressure on the military to address the problem reflected similar dynamics unfolding on campuses and workplaces across the country where women were organizing around the issue, including filing lawsuits against institutions for tolerating abuse.

One institutional difference, however, centered on the dependency of the military on female recruits during the long wars in Iraq and Afghanistan. Much like the World War II campaigns to recruit women into the war effort, the repeated deployments and overstretched military in the post-9/11 era necessitated a range of gender accommodations. In addition, reliance on an all-volunteer military brought changes to military culture itself. As psychologist and Major Jim Sardo described it, "if you don't take care of your soldiers and know how to keep them, and you're dependent on an all-volunteer Army, you're in a world of hurt." The roll-out of behavioral health programs and the move to incorporate feelings of vulnerability and helplessness into the warrior ethos were part of a distinctive feminizing of military culture.

Heightened attention to the problem of sexual assault led to more preventive measures, such as the Army's I.A.M. Strong Program, which included short videos linking the Soldier's Creed principle of "leaving no comrade behind" to bystander interventions in situations where other soldiers were being sexually harassed or threatened. Sexual assault programs made abuses suffered in the course of service more nameable and opened the door for victims to make claims on the system for treatment and in disability hearings. It also meant that victims were more likely to report. Indeed, Kimerling et al. (2007) conclude that VA policy regarding MST may be "the most comprehensive health policy response to sexual violence of any major US health care system" (p. 216).

The Tailhook and Aberdeen scandals of the 1990s were major catalysts in public demands to address the systematic nature of the problem (Lancaster, 1999; O'Neill, 1998; Violanti, 1996). Tailhook involved sexual incidents at a United States Navy and US Marine Corps convention in 1991 at a hotel in Las Vegas. More than 100 officers were charged with assaulting 83 women and 8 men over the three days of the conference. The Aberdeen scandal involved the United States Army and events at a Maryland training center in 1996. In the course of the investigation, 12 drill instructors were charged with sex crimes and 4 were sentenced to prison. These widely publicized scandals exposed the Armed Forces to widespread public criticism, and it became apparent that the military had a deeply rooted cultural problem (O'Neill, 1998).

Congress began passing bills on sexual assault prevention and reporting shortly after the Tailhook and Aberdeen scandals and even into the years of the draw down of the military, with many of the bills focused on better tracking of incidents (Department of Defense, 2018). Reports indicated that programmatic efforts were disappointing at best. A 2019 summary concluded that "the Department's scientific survey of the active duty force in Fiscal Year 2018 found that the estimated past-year prevalence (number of Service members endorsing an experience) of sexual assault increased, primarily for female service members ages 17 to 24." The survey found that the vast majority of sexual assaults were among younger service members of equal or similar rank and living in close proximity.

In her 2013 commentary in *Stars and Stripes*, Nancy Montgomery notes that the language and tone of outrage routinely expressed by military commanders mimes statements from 16 years prior, with each report seasoned with the same pledge to restore the trust of female service members: "Anything that might erode that trust is just not tolerable. We will maintain it, and we will enforce it. We will ensure that our people are treated with the human respect and dignity that they deserve."

## Institutional Pathologies

Much like the crisis around child sexual abuse in the Catholic Church, the military sexual assault crisis generated a range of diagnostic judgments concerning the etiology of the problem and prospects for meaningful reform. The challenge of untangling sexual harassment from normative practices in the military can be daunting. The maintenance of group cohesion in the military traditionally has relied on a hyper-masculine ethos, organized around eroticized and intensive male bonding. As a medium of male bonding, heterosexual jokes allow men to repress homoerotic feelings stirred by the intense camaraderie of war. The female Other also serves as receptacle for disallowed and externalized feelings of terror and vulnerability (O'Neill, 1998).

More than the posttraumatic stress disorder diagnosis itself, MST situates the source of pathology in military culture. Whereas PTSD narratives center on the emotional impact of combat or engagement with the enemy, military sexual trauma foregrounds pathogenic relationships within the institution itself. And, much like the incest narrative, which carried a critique of the patriarchal family, MST exposes the hypocrisy of military camaraderie presumably organized around the ethos of protection. Victims point out how fellow service members violate the Soldier's Creed and its mandate to protect your buddies and leave no comrade behind.

Clinicians working with female veterans report a recurring story of reluctance to acknowledge the impacts of sexual abuse. Many describe their struggles in getting women to feel entitled to their grievances. Rather than being angry, women are more apt to feel depressed and to downplay the effects of sexual assault. Military culture and the warrior identity require considerable capacity to "suck it up." Yet groups of women veterans have formed around the shared experience of sexual trauma (L. Daniels, personal communication, May 2, 2011).

At several workshops on MST that I attended, presenters described the identity crisis many female veterans experience after deployment. According to Nancy Sloan, the Women Veterans Program Manager at the Portland VA, "Many of them explain to me that they want a brother that will protect them. And they also want to be like a man." Sloan describes this ambivalence as a developmental process of self-discovery interrupted by the trauma of sexual assault. "A man will sexually abuse her," she goes on to say, "and everything that she dreamed of goes out the window and she's left without anything and really questioning her whole sense of self." Although they tended to downplay how warfare dehumanizes men and contributes to violent acting out, presenters did stress that sexual assault was a *political act*—an assault on the victim's gender and a tactic for preserving male bonds of camaraderie through the exclusion of women.

Many of the clinicians had undergone trainings to screen for MST after deployment and a number were also involved in treatment programs specializing in PTSD and MST. For these clinicians, the trauma story of female veterans—the Criterion A of the diagnosis—more often than not involved an incident of sexual assault that had been minimized, repressed, or simply endured until later symptoms of PTSD developed. As difficult as the struggle was to force the military and VA to address sexual assault in the military, MST had by 2010 become the signature trauma of female service members. Irene Fast, a VA psychologist, describes female veterans who endured horrific situations driving vehicles through areas under intense fire, picking up body parts after an explosion, which by any measure would seem traumatic. She explains that these disturbing scenes often arise in the course of evaluating for sexual assault.

Psychologist Jim Sardo talks with clinicians routinely at the VA about the new guidelines for MST, although most cases for female veterans are treated by female clinicians. In one session, he advises another VA psychologist as she prepares to deploy to Afghanistan, explaining that the commander ultimately makes the call on mental health assessments. But commanders are also aware of the potential political fallout of bad calls, Sardo adds. He tells a story to illustrate tensions that sometimes arise with commanders, but the story illustrates as well the two-sided aspects of military responses to sexual assault. While in Iraq, he had been asked to evaluate a soldier who was raped on her way to her deployment by a soldier from a different unit. She wanted to see someone from behavioral health about the rape but she also wanted to continue with her deployment. Sardo explains how her commander "had announced over an open radio that this Sergeant is asking for permission to get rape counseling." He goes on to explain how "600 guys in the unit were immediately informed. From there, lots of remarks, and the attention really made her more symptomatic." He describes his own distress as he attempts to support the soldier who is less and less able to function, his recommendation to the commander that she be evacuated for treatment, and the commander's refusal of the recommendation. The soldier then calls her mother stateside, who is furious and worried about her daughter and contacts the person in charge of sexual assault reporting in her region:

> What ended up happening was the person at the home base who was in charge of this program was the commander's wife. And when she heard about this commander who was keeping this poor rape victim in country, and found out that it was her husband, they dropped her off at my doorstep. Literally. They dropped her off unannounced and said, "we want

her out of the country in two days. Because this guy's wife called him up
and read him the riot act."

(J. Sardo, personal communication, May 5, 2011)

While the soldier's mother and the commander's wife could join forces in this
case, they drew on traditional obligations of good patriarchal leaders in relation to young women. The military asks a great deal of service members but
carries obligations in return to protect service members, including from abuse
in their own ranks. But another obligation is to maintain the fighting forces.
Sardo expresses some sympathy for commanders under pressure to keep the
mission going and for their tendency to resist investigations that they view as
bogging down the mission. The commander is under pressure from the gener-
als, who are under pressure from the executive branch.

Since MST refers to a complaint rather than a diagnosis, the assessment during military service centers on assault as a legal category with associated disciplinary actions, including the potential for dishonorable discharge and prison
sentences. In the military context, the victim has the right to file a complaint.
But not unlike sexual harassment in the workplace or domestic violence in the
home, power dynamics in the military make the exercise of such rights exceed-
ingly difficult. Most victims are diagnosed and treated through the VA system
following military service. As women enter the military in historically unprecedented numbers and are increasingly deployed "outside the wire" (beyond the
protection of forward operating bases), female service members move from
support roles to arenas of combat. Women service members, like their male
counterparts, carry home a range of war stories. Yet military sexual trauma
took center stage as the one story that summoned public interest during the US
wars in Iraq and Afghanistan (Lazare, 2011).

In one sense, the MST category carries the political ethos of the early PTSD
movement by situating psychiatric symptoms in the pathogenic context of warfare. Therapists often frame MST as analogous to incest in that it represents a
failure of paternal protectors and a violation of familial bonds. Nancy Sloan
speaks to this parallel: "They're [female soldiers] not safe at home, where
they're supposed to be safe with their 'brothers.' But they're not safe" (personal communication, April 2, 2011). The prototypical MST story exposes illusions behind the military as *pater familias*.

At the same time, the focus on betrayals of innocence in the MST story forti-
fies the familial model of the command structure in ways that mystify authority
relations in the military (Haaken & Palmer, 2012). Unlike good parents, officers have the job of getting the most out of their "assets." Effective commanders
express caring and concern for their units. But they also are in positions that
require getting young people to take enormous risks and to engage in forms of
violence that may violate internalized moral codes.

With MST as the most available container for the grievances of female
service members, less dramatic events fall below the threshold of public

interest. Non-traumatic sexual experiences, which also occur at a high frequency in the military, become more difficult to talk about. Indeed, military rules that make sex outside of marriage subject to disciplinary action cast a cloud of silence over everyday sex during deployment. Female and male service members alike spoke of the stress and loneliness of long deployments, combined with the intense camaraderie of working together. These dynamics intensify sexual feelings and longings, as well as assaultive acting out. Although military sexual trauma is difficult to expose, it may be more difficult to talk about the continuum of sexual experiences men and women have while on deployment. Media discussion routinely describes MST as the military's "dirty secret" ("The Military's Dirty Secret," 2012). As anthropologist Mary Douglas (1966/2002) so famously observed, "if we can abstract pathogenicity and hygiene from our notion of dirt, we are left with the old definition of dirt as matter out of place." Sex itself may be the dirty secret that can meet the light of day only when exposed as an impurity.

## Conclusions

This chapter focuses on war stories because these accounts are so highly associated with the PTSD diagnosis and the primary sites for studying breakdown under conditions of extreme stress. In drawing on my field work, I introduce feminist psychoanalytic modes of listening to these stories. Even elements of the prototypical soldier's story undergo repression as they are constructed through PTSD treatment protocols. The narrative structuring of PTSD for female veterans does bring betrayal by military culture into the syndrome. But the crisis routinely centers on a sexually chaste female soldier and her loss of innocence. Women's experiences in combat zones are stripped of their moral complexity, including conflict over military missions or their own personal engagement in warfare.

Clinicians bring their own cultural anxieties into the narrative structuring of complaints, including anxieties over what happens to young people when they go off to war. Like other neurotic symptoms, obsessive efforts on the part of clinicians to manage distress through PTSD protocols ultimately fail, in part because the reach of the control strategy exceeds its grasp. In the next chapter, I go deeper into a question that has dogged the PTSD movement from the start: how to take into account those vulnerabilities and problems that the person brings to a traumatic event. Evidence of over a century suggests that preexisting personality characteristics contribute to the clinical picture. But the PTSD field has had difficulty holding onto this part of the picture along with the idea that the disorder is a "normal response to an abnormal situation." As morally suspect disturbances, those carrying the diagnosis of personality disorder face higher hurdles in moving audiences with their tales of suffering.

# References

Alford, C. F. (1989). *Melanie Klein and critical social theory: An account of politics, art, and reason based on her psychoanalytic theory.* New Haven, CT: Yale University Press.

American Psychiatric Association. (2013). *Diagnostic and statistical manual of mental disorders (DSM-5).* Washington, DC: Author.

Brewin, C. R., Andrews, B., & Valentine, J. D. (2000). Meta-analysis of risk factors for posttraumatic stress disorder in trauma-exposed adults. *Journal of Consulting and Clinical Psychology, 68*(5), 748–766. https://doi.org/10.1037/0022-006X.68.5.748

Brewin, C. R., Lanius, R. A., Novac, A., Schnyder, U., & Galea, S. (2009). Reformulating PTSD for DSM-V: Life after Criterion A. *Journal of Traumatic Stress, 22*(5), 366–373. https://doi.org/10.1002/jts.20443

Brunner, J. (2000). Will, desire and experience: Etiology and ideology in the German and Austrian medical discourse on war neuroses, 1914–1922. *Transcultural Psychiatry, 37*(3), 295–320. https://doi.org/10.1177/136346150003700302

Burack, C. (2002). IV. Re-Kleining Feminist Psychoanalysis. *Feminism & Psychology, 12*(1), 33-38.

Caruth, C. (1991). Unclaimed experience: Trauma and the possibility of history. *Yale French Studies, Literature and the Ethical Question* (79), 181–192. Retrieved from JSTOR.

Cooper, D. (2001). *Psychiatry and anti-psychiatry.* London, UK: Routledge.

Davidson, J. R. T., & Foa, E. B. (1993). *Posttraumatic stress disorder: DSM-IV and beyond.* Washington, DC: American Psychiatric Press.

Department of Defense. (2018). *Annual report on sexual assault in the military.* Retrieved from Department of Defense website: https://int.nyt.com/data/documenthelper/800-dod-annual-report-on-sexual-as/d659d6d0126ad2b19c18/optimized/full.pdf#page=1

Dobbs, D. (2009). The post-traumatic stress trap. *Scientific American, 300*(4), 64–69.

Douglas, M. (1966). *Purity and danger: An analysis of concepts of pollution and taboo.* New York, NY: Routledge.

Frankl, V. E. (1976). *Man's search for meaning.* New York, NY: Pocket Books.

Freud, S. (1914/1957). *The standard edition of the complete psychological works of Sigmund Freud, volume XIV (1914–1918): On narcissism: An introduction.* (J. Strachey, Ed.). London, UK: The Hogarth Press.

Frueh, B. C., Hamner, M. B., Cahill, S. P., Gold, P. B., & Hamlin, K. L. (2000). Apparent symptom overreporting in combat veterans evaluated for PTSD. *Clinical Psychology Review, 20*(7), 853–885. https://doi.org/10.1016/S0272-7358(99)00015-X

Gilbert, S. M. (1983). Soldier's heart: Literary men, literary women, and the Great War. *Signs, 8*(3), 422–450. https://doi.org/10.2307/3173946

Good, B. J., Good, M.-J. D., Hyde, S. T., & Pinto, S. (2008). Postcolonial disorders: Reflections on subjectivity in the contemporary world. In *Postcolonial disorders* (pp. 1–40). Berkley, CA: University of California Press.

Haaken, J. (2013). *Guilty except for insanity: Maddening journeys through an American asylum* [Documentary]. Retrieved from www.guiltyexcept.com/sponsors

Haaken, J., & Palmer, T. (2012). War stories: Discursive strategies in framing military sexual trauma. *Psychoanalysis, Culture & Society, 17*(3), 325–333. https://doi.org/10.1057/pcs.2012.7

Herman, J. L. (1992). *Trauma and recovery: The aftermath of violence—From domestic abuse to political terror* (Rev. ed.). New York, NY: Basic Books.

Hurst, A. F. (1917). Observations on the etiology and treatment of war neuroses. *The British Medical Journal, 2*(2961), 409–414.

Kardiner, A. (1941). *The traumatic neuroses of war*. New York, NY: P. B. Hoeber, Inc.

Kimerling, R., Gima, K., Smith, M. W., Street, A., & Frayne, S. (2007). The Veterans Health Administration and military sexual trauma. *American Journal of Public Health, 97*(12), 2160–2166. Retrieved from http://empower-daphne.psy.unipd.it/userfiles/file/pdf/Kimerling%20R_%20-%202007.pdf

Kinzie, J. D., & Goetz, R. R. (1996). A century of controversy surrounding posttraumatic stress-spectrum syndromes: The impact on DSM-III and DSM-IV. *Journal of Traumatic Stress, 9*(2), 159–179. https://doi.org/10.1002/jts.2490090202

Kleinman, A. (2011). The art of medicine: The divided self, hidden values, and moral sensibility in medicine. *The Lancet, 377*(9768), 804–805. Retrieved from http://search.proquest.com.proxy.lib.pdx.edu/psycinfo/docview/858289175/117310B5D89545ABPQ/1?accountid=13265

Kleinman, A. (2012). Rebalancing academic psychiatry: Why it needs to happen—and soon. *The British Journal of Psychiatry, 201*(6), 421–422. http://dx.doi.org.proxy.lib.pdx.edu/10.1192/bjp.bp.112.118695

Koenen, K. C. (2007). Genetics of posttraumatic stress disorder: Review and recommendations for future studies. *Journal of Traumatic Stress, 20*(5), 737–750. https://doi.org/10.1002/jts.20205

Lancaster, A. R. (1999). Department of Defense sexual harassment research: Historical perspectives and new initiatives. *Military Psychology, 11*(3), 219–231. https://doi.org/10.1207/s15327876mp1103_1

Layton, L. (2015). Beyond sameness and difference: Normative unconscious processes and our mutual implication in each other's suffering. In D. Goodman & M. Freeman (Eds.), *Psychology and the other* (1st ed., pp. 168–188). Retrieved from www.oxfordscholarship.com/view/10.1093/acprof:oso/9780199324804.001.0001/acprof-9780199324804-chapter-11

Lazare, S. (2011, October 20). Military sexual assault and rape "epidemic." *Al Jazeera English*. Retrieved from www.aljazeera.com/indepth/features/2011/09/2011916112412992221.html

Levin, A. P., Kleinman, S. B., & Adler, J. S. (2014). DSM-5 and posttraumatic stress disorder. *Journal of the American Academy of Psychiatry and the Law Online, 42*(2), 146–158.

Lifton, R. J. (1985). *Home from the war: Vietnam veterans: Neither victims nor executioners*. New York, NY: Basic Books.

Litz, B. T., Stein, N., Delaney, E., Lebowitz, L., Nash, W. P., Silva, C., & Maguen, S. (2009). Moral injury and moral repair in war veterans: A preliminary model and intervention strategy. *Clinical Psychology Review, 29*(8), 695–706. https://doi.org/10.1016/j.cpr.2009.07.003

Loftus, E., & Ketcham, K. (1996). *The myth of repressed memory: False memories and allegations of sexual abuse* (Revised). New York, NY: St. Martin's Griffin.

MacLeish, K. (2018). On "moral injury": Psychic fringes and war violence. *History of the Human Sciences, 31*(2), 128–146. https://doi.org/10.1177/0952695117750342

Malik, M. L., & Beutler, L. E. (2002). The emergence of dissatisfaction with the DSM. In L. E. Beutler & M. L. Malik (Eds.), *Rethinking the DSM: A psychological perspective* (pp. 3–15). Washington, DC: American Psychological Association.

McNally, R. J. (2009). Can we fix PTSD in DSM-V? *Depression and Anxiety*, *26*(7), 597–600. https://doi.org/10.1002/da.20586

McNally, R. J., & Frueh, B. C. (2013). Why are Iraq and Afghanistan War veterans seeking PTSD disability compensation at unprecedented rates? *Journal of Anxiety Disorders*, *27*(5), 520–526. https://doi.org/10.1016/j.janxdis.2013.07.002

The Military's Dirty Secret. (2012, December 30). *The New York Times*. Retrieved from www.nytimes.com/2012/12/31/opinion/the-militarys-dirty-secret.html

Montgomery, N. (2013, July 7). After 2 decades of sexual assault in military, no real change in message. *Stars and Stripes*. Retrieved from www.stripes. com/news/after-2-decades-of-sexual-assault-in-military-no-real-change-in-message-1.229091

Nash, W. P. (2006). The spectrum of war stressors. In C. R. Figley & W. P. Nash (Eds.), *Combat stress injury: Theory, research, and management* (pp. 18–69). New York, NY: Routledge.

Nash, W. P., & Litz, B. T. (2013). Moral injury: A mechanism for war-related psychological trauma in military family members. *Clinical Child and Family Psychology Review*, *16*(4), 365–375.

Newman, L. M., & Schum, M. (1983). Factitious posttraumatic stress disorder. *American Journal of Psychiatry*, *140*(8), 1016–1019. Retrieved from http://ajp.psychiatry-online.org.proxy.lib.pdx.edu/doi/pdf/10.1176/ajp.140.8.1016

O'Neill, W. L. (1998). Sex scandals in the gender-integrated military. *Gender Issues*, *16*(1–2), 64–85. https://doi.org/10.1007/s12147-998-0016-y

Ozner, E. J., & Weiss, D. S. (2004). Who develops posttraumatic stress disorder? *Current Directions in Psychological Science*, *13*(4), 169–172. https://doi.org/10.2307/20182942

Patihis, L., Ho, L. Y., Tingen, I. W., Lilienfeld, S. O., & Loftus, E. F. (2014). Are the "memory wars" over? A scientist-practitioner gap in beliefs about repressed memory. *Psychological Science*, *25*(2), 519–530. https://doi.org/10.1177/0956797613510718

Russell, M. C., Schaubel, S. R., & Figley, C. R. (2018). The darker side of military mental healthcare part two: Five harmful strategies to manage its mental health dilemma. *Psychological Injury and Law*, *11*(1), 37–68. https://doi.org/10.1007/s12207-017-9311-9

Shatan, C. F. (1972, May 6). Post-Vietnam syndrome. *The New York Times*. Retrieved from www.nytimes.com/1972/05/06/archives/postvietnam-syndrome.html

Shay, J. (2003). *Odysseus in America: Combat trauma and the trials of homecoming*. New York, NY: Simon and Schuster.

Shay, J. (2014). Moral injury. *Psychoanalytic Psychology*, *31*(2), 182–191. https://doi.org/10.1037/a0036090

The Shay Moral Injury Center. (n.d.). Retrieved November 30, 2019, from Volunteers of America: Moral Injury website: www.voa.org/moral-injury-center

Southard, E. E. (1919). *Shell-shock and other neuropsychiatric problems*. Boston, MA: W.M. Leonard.

Spitzer, R. L., & First, M. B. (2005). Classification of psychiatric disorders. *Journal of the American Medical Association*, *294*(15), 1898–1900. https://doi.org/10.1001/jama.294.15.1898

Street, A. E., & Stafford, J. (2009). Military sexual trauma: Issues in caring for veterans. In *Iraq War clinician guide* (pp. 66–69). Retrieved from www.ce-credit.com/articles/101165/9-101165.pdf

Street, A. E., Vogt, D., & Dutra, L. (2009). A new generation of women veterans: Stressors faced by women deployed to Iraq and Afghanistan. *Clinical Psychology Review*, *29*(8), 685–694. https://doi.org/10.1016/j.cpr.2009.08.007

Tedeschi, R. G., & McNally, R. J. (2011). Can we facilitate posttraumatic growth in combat veterans? *American Psychologist*, *66*(1), 19–24.

van der Kolk, B. (2015). *The body keeps the score: Brain, mind, and body in the healing of trauma* (Reprint edition). New York, NY: Penguin Books.

Violanti, M. T. (1996). Hooked on expectations: An analysis of influence and relationships in the Tailhook reports. *Journal of Applied Communication Research*, *24*(2), 67–82. https://doi.org/10.1080/00909889609365442

Yehuda, R. (Ed.). (2006). *Psychobiology of posttraumatic stress disorders: A decade of progress, vol. 1071*. Hoboken, NJ: Blackwell Publishing.

# Chapter 2

# Trauma and Troubled Personalities

An anthem to the Merry Pranksters and road rebels of the 1960s, *One Flew Over the Cuckoo's Nest* celebrates impulses animating the highly masculinist beat generation. Published in 1962 and made into a film in 1975, Ken Kesey's tale of the asylum secured a lasting place in the social imaginary. Kesey was particularly attuned to psychological currents in American manhood. The crisis of the story unfolds as McMurphy, who maneuvered to get into the state hospital to escape jail time, charged with "too much fucking and fighting," discovers that most of his fellow patients entered the facility voluntarily. He comes to his own street diagnosis in summing up their troubles as insufficient assertions of manhood. Under the control of the repressed and repressive Nurse Ratched, the men on the ward choose to stay even when given the chance to leave. McMurphy launches his own subversive program to rehabilitate his fellow patients. He finds a prostitute to have sex with Billy, the boy suffocated by his overbearing mother, and instigates various ward insurrections. Chief, a Native American hospitalized for catatonia who emerges as the sentient ally of the rebellious McMurphy, emancipates himself from the control of Nurse Ratched at the film's conclusion. After the lobotomized McMurphy is wheeled onto the ward, mentally castrated for orchestrating a rebellion, Chief performs a mercy killing by smothering the tragic hero. Gathering up the strength within his massive frame, he then extracts a hydrotherapy machine from its plumbing fixtures and hurls it through a barred window of the day room. In the final scene, Chief jumps through the window casing and runs toward the Oregon hills, with a glorious sunrise over the Cascades signaling the dawn of a new era. For many poor and working-class men who hit the road, however, including Native American men, the highway to freedom remains illusory indeed.

In undertaking a documentary titled *Guilty Except for Insanity*, set at the same state hospital where *Cuckoo's Nest* was shot, I was particularly interested in the moral and political boundary between prisons and state hospitals—a boundary psychiatry regulates through its classification systems. The profession carries a long history of efforts to separate the truly mentally ill—the Billies who evoke sympathy as well as pity—and the McMurphies thought to be willfully defiant and deserving of jail time. But psychiatry confronts resistances on many levels. America, after all, loves its bad boys—a fixation that even 150 years of feminist campaigning has failed to successfully treat.

The critical psychiatry/anti-psychiatry movement of the 1960s and 1970s embraced some of these same romantic currents, seeing signs of societal rebellion in the rantings of the paranoid schizophrenic. PTSD proponents of the 1970s and 1980s carried variants of this ethos into their critique of diagnostic practices, but the movement accepted more of the premises of psychiatry and its role in demarcating distinctions between normal and abnormal behavior. There were a range of positions within the anti-psychiatry movement, but they shared a respect for diagnoses associated with deep disturbances. People exhibiting psychotic symptoms were cast as the Cassandras of the social order, tormented by apocalyptic visions of social breakdown and issuing warnings that fell below the threshold of audibility for normal people. PTSD advocates reclaimed the psychiatric dispossessed—the schizophrenics, suicidal depressives, and sociopaths— by building on the idea that disturbed people only appear to be mad. Their symptoms were a "normal response to an abnormal situation."

The PTSD movement confronted the hard limits of its campaign as advocates took up cases of people diagnosed with a personality disorder. Prisons hold vast numbers of traumatized people cast in ways that fall below the registers of public sympathies. These are cases where the mental disturbances are assumed to lie deep in the psyche and to occupy a region beyond the reach of psychiatry. Their profiles mark a moral boundary between those judged to be "mad" and those thought to be simply "bad." Prior to the fifth edition of the DSM, Axis II was the section of the manual listing personality disorders and developmental disturbances—conditions considered relatively unresponsive to treatment. Indeed, Axis II conditions became (and remain) the shorthand term for personality disorders, and particularly antisocial, narcissistic, and borderline disorders. The psychiatric boundary between these axes marking treatable and less treatable symptoms is in part an artifact of politics. Indeed, state laws intervene to adjudicate these diagnostic distinctions as the DSM-5 acknowledges. Although primarily written for clinicians, "DSM-5 is also used as a reference for the courts and attorneys in assessing the forensic consequences of disorders" (American Psychiatric Association, 2013, p. 25).

In this chapter, I look at how the PTSD diagnosis has straddled the moral and legal divide between treatable conditions and personality disorders, the sick and the despised. If the PTSD diagnosis is itself a symptom of a crisis in psychiatry, its incursion into the terrain of the personality disorders is where the crisis is most acute. These are morally inscribed diagnostic zones in psychiatry that carry a dark history. In taking up a genre of trauma stories associated with the personality disorders, I also return to the concept of *moral injury* as it is invoked to explain PTSD and why this concept fails to bridge politically charged distinctions between treatable and less treatable conditions. Gender dynamics emerge at these sites where competing diagnostic narratives determine the fates of troubled people as well.

In the years that followed the entry of PTSD into the DSM-III, civil and criminal courts emerged as the site for a new wave of psychiatric expertise. Legal scholar Alan Stone (Stone, 1993) offers an exalted assessment, as well as a caveat:

> The concept of PTSD has demonstrated an almost awesome capacity to rework the psychological narratives of life experience. From the Holocaust survivor to the incest survivor, PTSD offers a new frontier of explanation. It seems at first to provide a world of Manichaean moral certainty—evil people traumatize innocent victims, but of course it is not that simple, indeed the victimizers claim to have been victims of the abuser.
>
> (p. 35)

For Stone, this Manichean diagnosis lost its clarity as it entered the Machiavellian complexities of the courts. Defendants who are most effective in using the diagnosis for self-defense pleas, Stone sardonically observes, are those whose life histories present as testimonies to virtue.

Criminal laws throughout the United States codify distinctions between the "sociopath" (what the DSM lists as antisocial personality disorder) and those who are mentally impaired in a way that limits their ability to conform their behavior to the requirements of the law. As defense attorney Alex Bassos explains it,

> there is no doubt that if you are labeled with a personality disorder, you are going to have trouble at every turn through the system. These are people who are somehow thought to be willfully bad and treated as such.
>
> (personal communication, April 18, 2008)

Indeed, the distinction between Axis I and II disorders in the DSM-IV reflects an important boundary between medicine and the law. *Mental illnesses* are thought to operate beyond the person's control but nonetheless separate from concepts of personhood. Just as a person may suffer from tuberculosis, so too a person may suffer from schizophrenia. The *personality disorders*, on the other hand, are thought to be more fundamental to the person and paradoxically subject to the exercise of freedom of will. The prisons are full of people described as having made "bad choices" and punished on the basis of those choices. Although their legal files often include histories of neglect and abuse as well as trauma that result from poverty or living in desperate conditions, their cases confront a wall of exclusionary rules in the field of psychiatry.

## Guilty Except for Insanity

In the course of filming *Guilty Except for Insanity* (Haaken, 2013), I was interested in how patients themselves understood the diagnoses assigned to them in the course of their institutionalization. Among patients featured in the documentary, Alex A.—female identified at the time and now a transgender man—was the one most attuned to the symptom clusters at the border of Axis I (the treatable conditions) and Axis II (the less treatable). Moving with the labored gait of many patients on anti-psychotic drugs, he made his way into the visitors' room to meet me one morning after a group session— the first meeting since our interviews at the institution the year prior. Alex was accompanied by two female attendants, and he gestured to the beige, stackable plastic chairs where we could chat. After almost two years in a residential treatment facility, he had been sent back to the state hospital after throwing a cup through a window at his group home, shattering the glass. Although contesting the police account of what happened, he seemed resigned, even relieved, to return to this institution he knew all too well. His purple hair and retro silk shirt gave him a punkish look, notable in a setting where creating flair is no small feat. I put the bag of onion potato chips on the table, apologizing for my failure to fulfill his standard request for chips and soda. In bringing cherry Pepsi to the hospital that morning, I had forgotten that only factory-sealed plastic containers are allowed. I was asked to discard the Pepsi at the scanner because of the metal can. Alex shrugged in acceptance, seemingly satisfied with the puffy sack of chips that did make it through security.

As we talked about his recent re-admission to the hospital, Alex explained that there would be changes in the DSM-5 manual that could affect his treatment. At one of his Psychiatric Security Review Board hearings that I had attended, I discovered just how astute a reader of psychiatric nosology he could be. His psychiatrist told the Board that Alex had been misdiagnosed and that Alex had himself caught the clinical error. "She was actually the one who pointed this out to me that she does not and never did meet the criteria for bipolar disorder," the doctor testified authoritatively. Alex and the doctor agreed that he suffered from borderline personality disorder, which is often confused with bipolar disorder and particularly in young women exhibiting highly unstable moods. Although Alex had been diagnosed periodically with PTSD over the years, PTSD was now listed as the Axis I condition, alongside the new diagnosis of borderline personality.

Alex was particularly offended by common stereotypes of women in psychiatric hospitals as "drama queens." As a female patient with a reputation for disruptive behavior, Alex felt the frequent victim of this dismissive label. One day when we met for an interview, I noticed that he had what looked like a buzz cut. He told me the story of how he had pulled out his hair upon returning to the ward after a highly stressful psychiatric review hearing. The story included an account of how one of the staff got him to stop pulling out his hair. "It was just like that famous scene from *Good Will Hunting* where the teacher comes in and keeps saying over and over to the student who's freaking out, 'it's not your fault, it's not your fault.'" Looking intently into my eyes and leaning forward, he paused for dramatic emphasis. "It was just like that. The staff made me look at him and kept saying 'it's not your fault' until he got me to stop."

This question of whether "it's your fault" echoes in the heads of many patients, as well as throughout the institutions that confine them. Most patients at the hospital are assigned a dizzying array of diagnoses over the course of their institutionalization, from schizophrenia, schizoaffective disorder, and bipolar disorder, to various designations of "not otherwise specified" (NOS)— which means that the clinical picture is too murky to establish a stable diagnosis. But whatever the categories in patients' charts, the state statutes disallows use of the insanity plea in situations where a personality disorder is the primary diagnosis ("Effect of qualifying mental disorder guilty except for insanity," 2017). Legislative rules in Oregon—and in most states—bar these diagnoses in order to narrow the portal of entry into state hospitals through the insanity plea. Legal use of the plea, whether "guilty except for insanity" or "innocent by reason of insanity," requires that the presence of mental illness impaired the person's reasoning ability. According to the *Model Penal Code*, diagnoses that meet criteria for the insanity plea specify that "because of mental disease or defect the person is unable to either understand the implications of his/her actions or conform his/her behavior to the requirements of the law" (American Law Institute, 1961, Section 4.01). The exclusion of the personality disorders is based on the assumption that these conditions do not involve dysfunction in cognitive abilities and thus the person is presumed to have knowingly violated the law.

Yet the question of the *degree* of volitional choice that operates in any disorder has dogged the mental health field throughout its history. Psychology has produced an array of mental tests and measurements but considerable uncertainty remains over the extent of control *any person* possesses over their own behavior, including behaviors associated with psychiatric symptoms. Clinicians can make an educated guess as to whether the agoraphobic person is really able to leave the house without crippling anxiety or the depressed person has the capacity to get out of bed in the morning and go to work. But these clinical judgments ultimately rely on the patient's own subjective assessments of their motivations and states of mind.

## Mad or Bad: On Being Sick

Disputes over classification systems carry a long history, one that registers competing domains of disciplinary control—a theme taken up in Michel Foucault's (1975) *Discipline and Punish: The Birth of the Prison*. Concepts of mental derangement and madness date back to antiquity. But the idiom of mental illness—as a condition separate from personhood—emerged as central to modernity and medical thinking that worked its way into the courts. As Alex Bassos explains: "Beginning in the 19th century, the role of mental illness became increasingly recognized by the courts. There were people who had committed terrible crimes that we as a society could just not morally put through the criminal justice system" (personal communication, May 18, 2008).

Addictions and personality disorders continue to occupy an ambiguous classificatory boundary between mental illness and problems framed as voluntary and approached as disciplinary challenges. Medical explanations for some disturbing behaviors did represent an advance over religious interpretations. Epilepsy, for example, had for centuries been understood as a form of demon possession. So, too, alcoholism was considered a sign of degeneracy. Alcoholics Anonymous produced one of the most important shifts in public health thinking by reframing drunkenness as an illness rather than a character flaw. Growing up in the 1950s, I recall sitting at the kitchen counter with my mother after school, listening to Pastor Bob on the radio with his cautionary tales about drunks on skid row needing to be saved by grace. But it was AA that rewrote the scripts available to alcoholics through its claiming of the medical model, a movement that the field of psychiatry resisted for decades (Dean & Poremba, 1983).

The DSM-5 abandoned the axial system, placing the personality disorders in its own section and alongside sections grouping other conditions with correlated features. The aim was to move away from the damning associations of the Axis II cluster and to adopt a more politically neutral classification system. While introducing no substantive changes in the definitions or criteria for personality disorders, the DSM-5 committee created two clusters, with Cluster A constituted by sub-types of people that are more socially avoidant (paranoid, schizoid, schizotypal) and Cluster B grouping sub-types of people who tend to be highly disruptive and bothersome to others (antisocial personality disorder, borderline personality disorder, histrionic personality disorder, and narcissistic personality disorder). The B group, and particularly the antisocial personality disorder (ASPD) category, has generated the most political heat as the diagnosis is routinely used in the criminal justice system (Pickersgill, 2012; Trestman, 2014).

The campaign to move away from categorical and toward dimensional approaches to personality disorders failed, however, even though a DSM-5 sub-committee proposed "an alternative 'hybrid' model . . . to guide future research" (American Psychiatric Association, 2013, p. XIIII). Most of the controversy centers on scientific and clinical grounds for adopting either the dimensional or the categorical approach (Lynam & Vachon, 2012; Trull, 2011). But the implications of this distinction are as much political as they are methodological. Categorical approaches tend to magnify individual differences, whereas dimensional approaches tend to make commonalities more salient. Critical traditions in psychopathology lean more toward the dimensional than the categorical. Homosexuality, for example, has throughout much of the history of psychiatry been categorized as a perversion and symptom of psychopathy. Freud (1924/1959) implicitly adopted a dimensional approach, however, in arguing that "psycho-analysis enables us to point to some trace or other of a homosexual object choice in everyone" (p. 38). Gay rights advocates led a successful campaign to eliminate homosexuality as a disorder from the *Diagnostic and Statistical Manual* by presenting research findings drawing on this dimensional approach and establishing that homosexual orientation alone is not predictive of psychopathology. In the DSM edition published in 1973, homosexuality was described as an orientation along a continuum of normalcy (Drescher, 2015). This DSM reform grew from intense political pressure on the American Psychiatric Association, however, to confront how their system of classification operated as a cause rather than a cure for the troubles of gay people.

DSM proponents of the antisocial personality disorder (ASPD) diagnosis have attempted to untangle the category from images of the psychopath that circulate in popular culture. Although psychopathy is recognized in DSM-5, the term refers to a trait within the antisocial personality cluster. In an article in *Psychology Today*, Scott Bonn (Bonn, 2016) excitedly exclaims to the readers of this popular magazine the progress in diagnosing psychopaths:

> Approximately one-third of all prison inmates who are considered to be "antisocial personality disordered" (ASPD) meet the criteria of severe psychopathy specified in the fifth edition of the *Diagnostic and Statistical Manual of Mental Disorders* (DSM-5). For the very first time, the APA recognized psychopathy as a "specifier" of clinical antisocial personality disorder in the DSM-5, although psychopathy is still not an officially accepted clinical diagnosis. The recognition of psychopathy as a specifier of clinical ASPD by the APA follows nearly fifty years of research and debate.
>
> (para. 13)

Offering a less sanguine assessment of this history of debates, Martyn Pickersgill (2012) sardonically notes, "the ghost of the psychopath continues to haunt the corridors of the APA" (p. 546). This metaphor may be a way of acknowledging the guilt hovering over psychiatry's own role in perpetuating the personality disorder diagnoses—categories routinely applied in sentencing to rationalize long prison terms. Although a small fraction of prison inmates conforms to the Hollywood or DSM image of the psychopath, the evildoer driven by sadism and a singular desire to inflict suffering retains a strong hold on popular culture.

Personality disorders are both real and fictive, both based on observable patterns of behavior and enlisted to rationalize institutional control of people who are bothersome to others. Indeed, the personality disorders are among the most unreliable of diagnostic categories. This means that clinicians often disagree on whether they apply to a case at hand, even when presented with the same material. Whatever the validity of these diagnoses clinically, they operate within the American criminal justice system as a means of rationalizing severe and unequal sentencing practices.

As forensic psychologist Alexander Millkey describes the difference in the old DSM manual: "an Axis I diagnosis is something that a person *has*, like an illness, and an Axis II diagnosis is something that they *are*, 'I am this way'" (personal communication, February 1, 2009). Disturbing others more than feeling themselves as disturbed, those diagnosed with a personality disorder are notably among the loudest critics of psychiatric authority. Much like the McMurphy character in *One Flew Over the Cuckoo's Nest*, the person is often targeted as a troublemaker, particularly those diagnosed as antisocial, paranoid, or borderline personality. Even as they exhibit differing features, personality disorders are often recognizable clinically through their difficult relationships with authority figures, including therapists.

The personality disorder diagnoses involve establishing that the pattern is of a longstanding nature, typically dating back to adolescence or early childhood. (DSM-5 extends some of these categories into childhood diagnoses.) The criteria include an enduring pattern of behavior that "deviates markedly from the expectations of the culture" (American Psychiatric Association, 2013). This caveat is meant to alert clinicians to the risk of pathologizing cultural practices, although criteria allow considerable latitude for clinicians' judgments concerning the "expectations of the culture" and in deciding which deviations reach DSM thresholds.

Clinicians have a harder time agreeing on the personality disorders than on most of the other diagnoses, in part because the clinical judgments reflect the frustrations and prejudices of practitioners as much as they do objective clinical signs (Mellsop, Varghese, Joshua, & Hicks, 1982; Rogers, 2003; Spitzer et al., 2009). Like other people, clinicians vary in their levels of tolerance for rule-violators. Further, institutional confinement produces some of the very symptoms associated with the personality disorders. In *Asylums*, sociologist Erving Goffman (1961) paints a vivid portrait of the ways that institutionalized persons struggle to hold onto their humanity, whether furtively sharing a cigarette, "cheeking" their meds, or wandering off the ward. Yet institutionalized persons who question the rules are routinely labeled manipulative. One social worker at the Oregon State Hospital told me that when patients ask to see their charts—their legal right—the request is often framed by ward staff as evidence of manipulation, a clinical sign of a personality disorder.

If there is an affinity between personality disorders and posttraumatic stress disorder, it is in the political and forensic settings where experts establish their own relevance in adjudicating claims. PTSD advocates early on argued for excluding psychiatric history or preexisting conditions in establishing criteria for the diagnosis—a debate taken up in the last chapter. Whether in veterans' claims or in cases involving rape victims, "predisposition" was code for attributing responsibility to the character flaws of claimants, including responsibility for their own mental suffering (McNally, 2003; Scott, 1990). In the women's movement of the late 20th century, advocates pushed for the passage of laws that restrict testimony related to previous sexual history (Borgida & White,

1978). For close to a century, psychiatrists, whether behavioral, psychoanalytic, or biomedical in their orientation, held that victims of sexual assault or domestic abuse either masochistically sought out the abuse or were too weak psychologically to defend themselves. PTSD advocates played important roles in countering these sexist biases that ruled against women who "had a past." But this new diagnosis brought its own performance demands as the dramatic power of the event itself—its capacity to produce a complete mental breakdown in the victim—took center stage (Haaken, 2017).

Given that psychiatric history has been used to justify shifting responsibility from the traumatic event (and those who carried it out) to the sufferers themselves, it is not surprising that preexisting conditions related to PTSD represent a contested field of research (Brewin, Andrews, & Valentine, 2000). One of the ongoing dilemmas of mental health reformers centers on how to foreground the destructiveness of what has been endured, whether war or sexual assault, without compromising the position of survivors/victims in their capacities to testify to such effects. Persons with psychiatric histories are often cast as unreliable witnesses to their own suffering. Insistence on the essential goodness of trauma survivors was in reaction to a bitter history of locating the source of mental health problems in the psyches of victims, and particularly those victims with little social power.

## Military Madness

In explaining how good people can do bad things, trauma theorists often enlist the concept of *dissociation*—an idea that took hold in late 19th-century psychiatry but gained new vitality in the trauma movement of the late 20th century (Haaken, 1998). Dissociationists argue that memories of trauma are often isolated in a fragmented form in the psyche much like an encapsulated cyst. Bessel van der Kolk (2000) cites Freud in explaining the relationship between repressed memory and acting out:

> Despite having abandoned the central problem of dissociation in response to trauma, Freud kept being fascinated with the issue of the compulsion to repeat it. In "Remembering, Repeating, and Working Through" Freud claimed that if a person does not remember, he is likely to act out.
>
> (p. 242)

The early PTSD movement showed how normal people could, under situations of extreme stress, develop symptoms that mimicked severe mental illness or a personality disorder. The concept of dissociation achieved wide currency in the 1990s because it established the trauma survivor as rational and morally capable, on the one hand, and severely damaged, on the other. The more disturbed the person's behavior, many trauma therapists reasoned, the more likely this behavior registered the effects of horrific past abuses. Violent veterans who got into bar fights or assaulted their partners in a fit of rage—key indicators of many personality disorders—were cast as enacting battle scenes in dissociated states (Bremner & Marmar, 2002). The dissociation, much like the concept of mental illness, created a conceptual bridge between forms of behavior that violate social norms—such as reckless or violent behavior—and the motivational states and attributes that make up the person. Memory of a traumatic event was believed to be compartmentalized in mind and separated from consciousness, only to emerge and overtake the person when a current situation triggered the memory and the dissociative defense broke down. While dissociation is a valid concept, trauma therapists built an entire theoretical edifice around its presumed use as a psychological defense against disturbing memories. Therapists tended to deny their own active roles in the dramas that unfolded around clinical excavation of disturbing scenes from the past (Haaken, 1998).

Since World War I, therapists have brought trauma into the clinical picture to elicit greater sympathy for those accused of crimes in both military and civilian settings. Psychiatrist Norman Camp (2015), author of *US Army Psychiatry in the Vietnam War*, a military psychiatry textbook, describes the intense controversies within this sub-field of medicine during the last half of the Vietnam War. In his review of lessons to be learned from the Vietnam War, Camp argues that the psychiatric categories available to clinicians were woefully inadequate in explaining the complex and situational array of disturbances displayed by the troops. Camp also takes up the politics of diagnosis. He claims that psychiatrists were pressured to diagnose soldiers on a large-scale basis under various personality disorder labels—an intervention that relieved the military of responsibility for service members' problems because of the widely shared assumption that these disorders are deeply rooted character problems.

The posttraumatic stress disorder campaign gathered support in response to the use of Axis II diagnoses as a basis for dishonorable discharge from the military. As mental health services were slashed and mass incarceration became a feature of late 20th-century America, progressive clinicians sought refuge for patients in the expansion of the trauma diagnoses (Jones & Wessely, 2007; Scott, 1990). Indeed, the development of special courts for veterans draws on the assumption that veterans' military trauma can lead to criminal behavior after a tour of duty—and that society has an obligation to provide supportive services to these veterans rather than jail or prison time (McCormick-Goodhart, 2012; Slattery, Dugger, Lamb, & Williams, 2013; Walls, 2010).

In the case of Robert Bales, the infantryman who carried out one of the worst atrocities in recent US military history, his legal team initially pursued a PTSD defense, describing his dissociated state on the night when Bales left his compound and murdered 16 civilian Afghanis in a nearby village. "Part of PTSD is dissociation," explains Charles Golden, a psychologist who wrote a report on Bales for the defense. He goes on to describe the phenomenon of depersonalization associated with dissociated states. "The person feels like he's watching himself or outside himself—he's not himself. And head trauma—we don't have a lot of research on that—but head trauma may exacerbate that tendency to dissociate when under stress" (as cited in Vaughan, 2015, XI para. 3). The drama that unfolds in media reports echoes some of the same psychological formulations that gained currency in the case of Captain Calley, who assassinated 22 unarmed villagers during the Vietnam War in the My Lai massacre. Calley was evaluated by a number of psychiatrists who concluded that the violence was the result of a "breakdown in repression"—the release of pent-up aggression as his psychic armor cracked (Anderson, 1972). Another clinician working for the Calley defense draws a similar clinical picture: "an over-inhibited personality structure fraught with internal conflict between impulses and repressive forces is sharply etched" (Anderson, 1972, p. 8A). Prior to the trauma therapy movement of the 1990s, psychodynamic therapists focused more on repression than dissociation as a mode of defense (see Haaken, 1998). While these constructs share certain features, repression involves more emphasis on intrapsychic conflict—for example, sadistic impulses and their defensive elaborations. Dissociation, on the other hand, tends to be understood as a defense against an *external* threat.

Bales ultimately made a deal with the prosecution to avoid the death penalty. Although he had been deployed four times and suffered traumatic brain injury in addition to witnessing the death of fellow soldiers, there was no single scene of trauma that would justify the PTSD diagnosis. With his history of fighting and heavy drinking, illegal securities transactions as a trader before entering the military, use of illicit drugs, and the cold-blooded murder of Afghani villagers, including shooting at close range women and small children, Robert Bales fell too deep into the personality disorder terrain to find redemption through psychiatry.

Although the madness and immorality of the wars in Iraq and Afghanistan figured prominently in public discourse over the atrocity, as it had in media coverage of the My Lai massacre during the Vietnam War, the forces that produced these monstrous soldiers ultimately eluded the instruments of military psychiatry. Dissociated states may indeed represent a combustible mix of adaptive and maladaptive defenses for the fighting forces—the two-edged sword of combat psychology. Former Secretary of Defense Robert S. McNamara offers a more apt metaphor for this condition in describing "the fog of war." McNamara defines the fog of war as meaning that "it's beyond the ability of the human mind to comprehend all the variables. Our judgment, our understanding, are not adequate. And we kill people unnecessarily" (as cited in Wead, 2015, p. 70).

Lost in this same fog of war are clear lines for assigning moral responsibility when warriors go berserk. The Geneva Convention after World War II codified into international law constraints on the use of violence, and particularly in treatment of civilians and prisoners of war. Service members are trained in what the military terms the Law of War, which includes Rules for Engagement (ROE), for example that the violence be proportionate to the magnitude of the threat and has the aim of eliminating the enemy. The rules require fighters to avoid causing unnecessary suffering. Yet the terrain on which many battles are fought cast a moral fog over how many of the rules are carried into practice. Unlike the legal cases that forced the Catholic Church to acknowledge responsibility for sexual abuse carried out by priests and the trauma suffered by their victims, war crimes carried out by service members rarely involve indictments against commanders. As Jeremy Dunnaback (2015) notes, US military criminal law offers considerable legal protection for commanders in the prosecution of war crimes. He also explains how wars carried out by the US military since Vietnam have been fought more often by small units of fighters than by large brigades. These small mobile units under the direct control of lower-ranking officers tend to be located in outposts removed from the larger command structure of the military. They cultivate tight bonds among fighters—a social situation that can produce violent acting out as well as camaraderie. For soldiers such as Bales, the question of whether he suffered from PTSD or antisocial personality disorder obscures this broader issue of how the theater of war becomes a stage for what McNamara terms "unnecessary killing."

The trauma movement organized around a shared commitment to expose psychic injuries habitually shut out of public view. It was a call for social justice, although the call rested heavily on establishing a wide class of experiences "outside of the normal" that led to disguised symptoms of trauma. Holocaust survivors were the focus of some of the early PTSD formulations, although diagnosticians immediately confronted the limits of their own categories (Lifton, 1980). As Katarzyna Prot (2010) notes in summarizing mental health literature on Holocaust survivors, "most authors consider the diagnosis of PTSD to be insufficient to describe the survivors' mental health problems" (p. 62). In taking up the debate over whether the Holocaust was representable, whether the scale of its horrors could be adequately represented given the limits of human language, Fred Alford (2009) explains how the question of how to talk about the effects of the Holocaust entered PTSD discourse as a "crisis of witnessing"—a crisis bound up in how expertise is enlisted to contain aspects of human history that seem utterly uncontainable. Alford adds that "PTSD is a psychological diagnosis which a few psychoanalysts, and a larger number of literary critics, have attempted to turn into a category of history" (p. 10).

More than Holocaust survivors, the fighters in various American war zones have served on the front lines of professional battles over trauma and the lessons of military history. As Ben Shephard (2003) concludes in his history of PTSD, public discourse on the psychiatric effects of combat have alternated between denial and exaggeration. The rhetorical convention of a hidden disturbance is used by both sides, whether in the anti-war imagery of veterans as walking time bombs or conservative charges that anti-war protesters are crypto-communists or subversives (Scurfield, 2006; Shay, 2003).

For the PTSD movement, aggressive or antisocial behaviors that resulted in dishonorable discharges for thousands of Vietnam War veterans could be portrayed as re-enactments of horrific battle scenes. Veterans groups have for decades challenged the military's use of Regulation 635–200, Chapter 5–13: "Separation Because of Personality Disorder." The Department of Veterans Affairs does not provide medical care to soldiers dismissed with a personality disorder, nor are these soldiers eligible for disability or other benefits. In July 2007, the House Veterans' Affairs Committee held a hearing concerning charges that the Defense Department was wrongfully discharging service members and denying benefits on the basis of this diagnosis.

## The Troubles of Military Psychiatry

The history of PTSD is often told through a trajectory of war-related clinical precursors—the 17th-century condition of *nostalgia*, the 19th-century *soldier's heart*, World War I *shell shock*, *battle fatigue* and *war neurosis*, and *neuropsychiatric disorders* during World War II. But it is instructive to approach PTSD as part of a reform movement within psychiatry in response to the use of personality disorders as disciplinary diagnoses. Rather than a traumatic event, PTSD can take the form of behavior that crosses a tense line in authorized use of violence under the intense stress of combat. Military clinicians note that features of both narcissistic and antisocial personality disorder symptoms *are functional* in war zones (J. Sardo, personal communication, June 8, 2011). Among the symptoms of both narcissistic and antisocial conditions is the tendency to treat people as instrumental objects and to lack empathy. Yet this same reasoning applies to therapists working within the military. Clinicians in Afghanistan describe their jobs as getting more value out of "military assets." Wars are built on instrumentality and the subduing of normal moral responses even as they require self-discipline and adherence to codes of military conduct.

The diagnoses assigned to breakdowns in functioning—whether labeled a character flaw or an effect of trauma—register the differing political stances of mental health professionals serving in the military as well as the institutional pressures they confront (Shephard, 2003). In their history of German psychiatry and the military, Kloocke, Schmiedebach, and Priebe (2005) describe how both World Wars were sites for re-conceptualizing psychic trauma as a factor in mental disorders. The wars provided psychiatry the opportunity to study emotional breakdown on a massive scale and to offer assessments on the role of character flaws in those breakdowns—a stance widely held by psychiatrists on both sides of these conflict.

German and Austro-Hungarian psychiatrists played notably leading roles during the Great War in generating the classification systems routinely enlisted to triage symptomatic soldiers. In the early phase of the war, psychiatric casualties in Germany were small, with diagnosed war neurotics under 5 percent (Kloocke et al., 2005). Jose Brunner (2000) describes the rise in more dramatic debilitating symptoms with the transition from military assaults to trench warfare in the winter of 1914–1915 and a corresponding expansion of characterological diagnoses. The distinction between neurologists and psychiatrists emerged as a morally charged border separating cases where symptoms were attributed to a traumatic shock to the nerves versus those cases thought to be more psychological, involving a lack of "will or desire" (Brunner, 2000).

Psychological screening and training of troops during World War I, along with the "forward psychiatry" model of short-term interventions in the form of a few days of rest and reassurance close to the front, seemed adequate early on in keeping pace with the military mission. But as the war dragged on, commanders in Britain, France and Germany turned to psychiatrists to manage the increasing numbers of soldiers either unable or unwilling to fight. Psychiatrists were enlisted to manage the growing problem of "battle fatigue." The difference between battle fatigue, which registered the limits of human endurance, and the more judgmental category of "war neuroses," reflected military doctors' own frustrations with the enormity of their task. The variability and range of symptoms clearly exceeded the tonics administered under the "three-hots-and-a-cot" treatment. Yet the commanders tended to view most of these conditions as breakdowns in military discipline. As Kloocke et al. (2005) suggest in reflecting back on this history, "discipline and fighting morale in the Army were jeopardized by the quasiinfectious spreading of the so-called 'war neuroses'" (p. 44). The spike in psychiatric cases as wars drag on for years has been documented throughout history, including in the Vietnam War (Cavenar & Nash, 1976; Hyams & Wignall, 1996).

Beyond the fate of soldiers, the professional fates of psychiatrists themselves were on the line. During both World War I and II, psychiatrists acquired authority through their reports from the front, many of which drew conclusions from personal observations in field hospitals. But beyond the question of what was wrong with soldiers who were no longer able or willing to fight, disputes over diagnosis served as the crucible for competing claims around professional authority. The British journal *Lancet* was particularly important in advancing the scientific legitimacy of military psychiatrists. A series of papers throughout the war years describes the diagnostic work of clinicians behind the front lines, complete with scientific tables listing categories separating types of war neurotics. A loose consensus developed around a personality type predisposed to breakdowns—those with a "weak spot in the personality" (Roberts-Pedersen, 2012). This attribution absolved both doctors and commanders of responsibility for the breakdown of soldiers, even as it opened space for acknowledging vulnerabilities not born of mere lack of discipline. But just as illness is not the fault of the person inflicted with the malady, the theory of a "weak spot" in the personality undermined the military's assertions that soldiers acted out of willful disobedience. Ideas around inheritable traits or inborn weaknesses tend to have a conservative cast, but they can also be enlisted to challenge claims of willful misconduct.

Whatever the weak spots that produced breakdowns, military doctors tended to frame such cases as the result of desperate efforts on the part of soldiers to comply with military commands. Some psychiatrists saw their role as educating commanders and the general public on the horrors of war, and particularly of trench warfare. Sir Grafton Eliot Smith and Tom Hatherly Pear (1917), authors of *Shell Shock and Its Lessons*, argue that the strongest and bravest soldiers are those who break down after having pushed themselves to the limits of human endurance. "Their strength of mind and body has been demonstrated over and over again, yet at last they have broken down" (p. 20). They stress the variability of psychiatric cases and how many breakdowns are produced by the horrific conditions of warfare rather than constitutional weakness. Infantrymen continue to be at the highest risk for psychiatric casualties, particularly after from three to six months of combat (J. Sardo, personal communication, June 5, 2011). With growing war-resistance alongside psychiatric casualties during the final years of the war, doctors were under increased pressure to separate the "hereditarily weak" and the "hearty soldier" and to locate their differential breaking points:

> It is, of course, unquestionable that in a large army there must be many soldiers with tainted family histories; and it is probably equally certain that such factors play some part in determining the greater susceptibility of certain men to shock. But it would be a gross misrepresentation of the facts to label all the soldiers who suffer from mental troubles as weaklings. The strongest man when exposed to sufficiently intense and frequent stimuli may become subject to mental derangement.
>
> (Smith & Pear, 1917, p. 36)

By World War II, a more humanitarian approach to diagnosis emerged in military psychiatry. Fear was routinely acknowledged and incorporated into codes of conduct. But soldiers were also expected to overcome fear. Doctors held little control over the conditions of the fight, but they did exercise some control over the fighters themselves. As historian Roberts-Pedersen (2012) describes the psychiatric situation of soldiers during World War II, border tensions arose between military psychiatry and military discipline:

> A tension thus emerged in the medical literature, which vacillated between sympathy for the suffering of fighting men (and concomitant speculations on the possibility of traumatic combat experience being independently causative) and an insistent avowal of the explanatory value of predisposition. . . . For predisposed individuals, even being "blown up" might be a welcome climax to a series of horrifying experiences upon which the patient can project his troubles, in the same way as the hysteric projects his external distress on to a physical injury.
>
> (p. 321)

While psychiatry played an important role in registering the psychological toll of warfare, diagnoses such as shell shock and battle fatigue had narrowed the focus to direct physical impacts and bio-physiological explanations. These "impact" diagnoses obscured the element of *resistance to military discipline* expressed in symptoms—a dynamic not lost to military critics of the "war neuroses" (Scurfield, 2006). As a psychiatric category based on the idea of repressed internal conflict, war neurosis admitted conflict over the war itself. Throughout much of the history of military psychiatry, the protection of emotionally distressed service members rested on establishing that their failure to follow commands was the result of sheer physical exhaustion.

## War Psychiatry and Psychoanalysis

As reports circulated in Vienna of brutal treatment of soldiers by army doctors, Freud was called before the Austrian War Ministry to give expert testimony. Introduced in 1919, his testimony was a defense of psychoanalytic treatment of war neurosis and a repudiation of the method of administering electrical shock to emotionally ill soldiers to prod them back into active duty. Reports of mental breakdown and suicides following treatments, and even lethal doses of shock, raised disturbing questions about the psychiatric management of hospitalized soldiers. In challenging the prevailing method of treatment, Freud (1921) suggested that soldiers' symptoms told an unconscious story of visceral struggle and heroic defeat. He explained how symptoms such as paralysis were a means of psychically escaping an unbearable conflict between the command to kill and deeply internalized moral prohibitions against such commands, a conflict exacerbated by "the ruthless suppression of his personality by his superiors" (pp. 212–213). Freud commented that:

> Only the smallest proportion of war neurotics were malingerers; the emotional impulses which rebelled in them against active service and drove them into illness were operative in them without becoming conscious to them. They remained unconscious because other motives, such as ambition, self-esteem, patriotism, the habit of obedience and the example of others, were to start with more powerful until, on some appropriate occasion, they were overwhelmed by the other, unconsciously-operating motives.
>
> (p. 213)

Beyond defending the psychoanalytic method on humanistic grounds, Freud was making a political intervention. Rather than attributing war neurosis to the problem of "shell shock" or the assaults suffered at the hands of the enemy, Freud focused on problems of authority on the home front. Massive desertions and active resistance became widespread among soldiers on both sides of the war during its final years, and psychiatrists were summoned to separate the malingerers and the war resisters from the truly ill. It is likely that many soldiers *were* consciously resisting or malingering through their symptoms, if only from sheer exhaustion or "combat fatigue." Freud stopped short of defending those who consciously refused to return to duty. But he did offer, through the concept of unconscious motivation, an escape clause that preserved the ideal of duty, honor, and patriotism even as it registered the power of resistance to such dictates. The irony in this psychoanalytic line of interpretation is that soldiers were only protected to the extent that such motives remained unconscious. Once rebellion became a conscious motive, however, the war-injured was forced to make a conscious choice: resist the war and face court martial or return to duty.

Siegfried Sassoon, a poet and decorated lieutenant in the British Army, won an honored place in history as among those few officers who resisted. After being wounded in action and evacuated for treatment and convalescence, Sassoon refused to return to duty. In a letter sent to his commanders and read in the House of Commons in July 1917, Sassoon stated the reasons for his decision:

> I am making this statement as an act of wilful defiance of military authority because I believe that the war is being deliberately prolonged by those who have the power to end it. I am a soldier, convinced that I am acting on behalf of soldiers. I believe that the war upon which I entered as a war of defence and liberation has now become a war of aggression and conquest. . . . I have seen and endured the sufferings of the troops and I can no longer be a party to prolong these sufferings for ends which I believe to be evil and unjust.

Sassoon expected to be court-martialed as a result of his public protest and refusal to return to duty. But fellow poet Robert Graves intervened on his behalf and convinced commanders that Sassoon suffered from shell shock and required psychiatric treatment rather than military discipline. He was treated at Craiglockhart war hospital by William Rivers—a military doctor and advocate of the psychodynamic "talking cure."

Throughout the World War II era, psychoanalysts held a leading role in diagnosing the maladies of combat (Leys, 2000; Miller & Miller, 1940; Shephard, 2003). The literature on trauma in the 1940s and 1950s followed in the wake of the displacements caused by war, where the work of Rene Spitz and Anna Freud on orphaned children ushered in the psychoanalytic movement toward object relations theory—an approach that departed from the classical Freudian focus on drives and ego defenses against them to a model that views human nature as attachment-seeking. The term "object" in this tradition refers to representations of people or parts of people that contribute to the formation of the psychological self and its sources of psychic stability and instability.

The object relations emphasis on early attachments and trauma associated with early losses resonated with the experiences of psychoanalytic theorists, many of whom had lost their own "mother country" through the displacements of war (Zaretsky, 2005). Ronald Fairbairn (1943) describes the traumatic rupture accompanying the infant's separation from the mother's body and entry into the world: "any post-natal experiences which provokes separation anxiety will in some measure assume the emotional significance of the original birth trauma" (p. 276). In this passage, taken from his essay on war neuroses, Fairbairn exclaims that the horrors of warfare awakened powerful terrors and dependencies of early life. While *birth trauma* never achieved legitimacy in most psychoanalytic traditions, Fairbairn was perhaps correct at the metaphorical level in framing the existential states of soldiers and their profound sense of emotional abandonment. Yet the metaphor also expressed a form of institutional defense in psychoanalysis itself around dependency on "maternal objects." As Fred Alford (2018) suggests in his review of psychoanalytic approaches to trauma, object relations theorists no less than the classical Freudians tended to view human development as a process of progressive capacities for separation and individuation. The longing to be held like an infant—the wounded soldier's anguished cry for his mama—represented a "regression in the service of the ego," but a regression none the less.

This tendency to pathologize dependency was notably pronounced in Fairbairn's (1943) diagnostic formulations. Indeed, his assessments of troubled soldiers anticipated the routine use of "dependent personality disorder" as a basis for discharge during the Vietnam War. This diagnosis encompasses a range of situations and behaviors, including situations where soldiers refuse to obey orders but in a way that is not openly defiant. In describing cases he treated in military hospitals, Fairbairn concludes that "like many a physically disabled soldier, the neurotic soldier wants to go home because he is ill." In reality, Fairbairn adds, "he is ill because he craves to go home. . . . It is impossible, therefore, to draw any real distinctions between the war neuroses and 'homesickness'" (p. 184). His explanation for why some soldiers break down while others withstand the rigors of military life centers on what he views as a failure to individuate and the soldier's infantile dependencies, which interfere with group bonding. As evidence, Fairbairn notes how often wounded soldiers cry out for their mothers.

One of the symptoms of a personality disorder is unresponsiveness to treatment—a symptom that can be as much a condition of the doctor as it is the patient. In apparent frustration, Fairbairn exclaims, "what these people really need is not a psychotherapist but an *evangelist*" (Fairbairn, 1943, p. 186). And he may have been correct in admitting of the limits of his own powers to get soldiers back on their feet.

Unlike Fairbairn, many psychoanalysts during this era did produce more complex understandings of war neurotics and sometimes more compassionate portrayals. Yet, much like the Great War, World War II became a battleground where psychoanalysts fought for legitimacy. The American psychoanalyst Carl Menninger (1948) declared a victory for psychiatry through the war effort: "Psychiatry struggled from the rear seat in the third balcony to finally arrive in the front row at the show" (p. vii). That "show" was the wider world of civil society and post-war adjustment beyond psychiatry's traditional role in institutions for the insane and military hospitals.

*Let There Be Light*, a film directed by John Huston and commissioned by the United States Army, exemplifies this post-war enlightened position of psychoanalytic psychiatry. The documentary includes moving portrayals of emotionally broken soldiers struggling to awaken from battlefield nightmares and face the terror that lingers in the form of debilitating symptoms. The progressive ethos of the film lies in its refusal to gloss over these effects of war. Indeed, the raw emotional vulnerability of the featured veterans led the Department of Defense to censure the film for decades after its completion. Yet the denouement offers a cheerily reassuring assessment of post-war recovery and climaxes in an exalted tribute to the powers of modern psychiatry. Doctors pronounce the men cured and ready to return to civilian life, no less hearty than the day they joined the good fight.

Not unlike other military clinicians, psychoanalysts during both world wars oriented their treatments in alignment with the war effort (Shephard, 2003; J. P. Wilson, 1994; M. Wilson, 1993). While insisting that every man has his breaking point, psychoanalysts shared the view of commanders that the aim of treatment is to get soldiers to return to duty. Once unconscious resistance to war was made conscious, as Freud's approach to the talking cure would suggest, further resistance carried the soldier from the protective category of war neurotic to the prosecutable class of malingerers—one of the characteristics of the personality disorders. For the troubled soldier, the distinction between conscious malingering and unconscious conflict was central to the diagnosis—and to the fate of the soldier.

## The Soul of the Soldier: Moral Injuries

Two prototypical approaches to trauma have survived the many eras of contestation over war neurosis, both of which were revisited by PTSD proponents in remapping the clinical picture for personality disorders in the late 20th century. One approach, rooted in the behavioral traditions (where psychiatry stays as close to biology as possible), understands neurosis as the result of an over-excited nervous system. The second, rooted in psychodynamic traditions, approaches the symptoms as an existential crisis in meaning or a rupture in self-object relations—the relative balance of nurturing versus persecuting representations ("bad objects") of others that inhabit the internal world.

Both approaches find pathways into areas of mind concealed from consciousness and both have ways of linking symptoms on the surface with a less observable substrate of mental processes. The behavioral approach—which encompasses a number of separate schools of thought—argues that warfare can produce personality changes through conditioning that affects the autonomic nervous system. Just as Russian experimental psychologist Ivan Pavlov showed how dogs would salivate at the sound of a bell paired with food and then continue to salivate when they heard that bell, soldiers returning from combat are conditioned to respond to stimuli as though there is still a war going on. This approach is often enlisted in military contexts, where the metaphor of voltages is used to explain the "rewiring" of the brain. The warrior running on 220 volts returns to a civilian world operating on 110 volts and everything feels unbearably slow (J. Sardo, personal communication, June 8, 2011). Like an addict, warriors seek out excitement—bar fights, speeding, drugs—to reset their brain physiology. The second approach—drawing on psychoanalytic principles—focuses on a moral or relational crisis produced by participating in warfare (Lifton, 1985; Shay, 1994). From this perspective, antisocial behavior registers a rupture in the capacity of the person to enlist internal "good objects" as the internalized representations of attachment figures. The breakdown in functioning following exposure to an overwhelming event is thought to be the result of a failure in the capacity for holding in mind and making use of connections with others.

Although some scholars note spikes in criminal behavior among veterans after wars (Archer & Gartner, 1992), other scholars conclude that the association between military service and crime is mediated by a complex range of factors (Culp, Youstin, Englander, & Lynch, 2013; Elbogen et al., 2012). The Department of Defense tracking data on incarceration rates among veterans documents a steady decline in rates from 1978 to 2012 (Lawrence, 2015). Reduced incarceration rates are also attributed to the rise of veterans' courts around the United States that allow more leniency for veterans in alternative sentencing.

PTSD holds special appeal for defense attorneys in veterans' criminal cases because the diagnosis is more apt to invite the sympathies of juries. The diagnosis offers a strategy for separating veterans from "ordinary criminals." Attorney Marcia Shein (2010) offers this counsel:

> The use of experts may be particularly powerful in explaining to the judge (or jury) how the PTSD affected a particular defendant's actions in order to make him or her less culpable. The expert may help distinguish the defendant before the court from the hundreds of other defendants who appear before the court asking for downward departures and variances.
>
> (p. 49)

For Vietnam veterans seeking services from VA clinics, the PTSD category provides a medical pathway in reframing disruptive behavior. Rather than outlaws, violent veterans are cast as reenacting the trauma of war, of fighting displaced enemies on their return (McCormick-Goodhart, 2012). Whether dishonorably discharged for aggressive behaviors or getting into bar fights after deployment, veterans found a more sympathetic response when their troubles were interpreted as re-enactments of nightmarish battle scenes.

During the Vietnam War, psychiatric casualties were low—under 2 percent—in part because troubled soldiers were discharged under disciplinary codes

(J. Sardo, personal communication, June 8, 2011; Camp, 2015). The Vietnam Veterans of America (VVA) filed two lawsuits in 2008 against branches of the military for discharging service members under personality disorder codes. The lawsuits, based on records obtained under the Freedom of Information Act, claimed that there was a pervasive pattern of commanders directing military psychologists to assign a diagnosis of personality disorder in order to get rid of soldiers identified as either troubled or troublesome. Further, the use of the diagnosis was grounds for denying benefits to service members. The label of dishonorable discharge associated with the psychiatric evaluation carries serious and lasting effects on veterans' employment record. The protocols for making the diagnosis have tightened since the suit was settled, although tensions remain over how boundaries are drawn between therapeutic and disciplinary use of psychiatric diagnoses (Leroux, 2015).

The struggle among clinicians over the degree of responsibility the military carries for symptomatic veterans has shifted toward greater recognition of the "moral injuries" of war—a concept taken up in the previous chapter. The term has acquired currency among progressive clinicians in extending the reach of war trauma into the personality disorders. While going beyond mechanistic stress models, the idiom of moral injury relies heavily on an impact model. The injury is conceptualized as a result of an external force, although the condition is often described as a "hidden injury of war" (Nash & Litz, 2013).

William Nash and Britt Litz (2013) have been leading voices in gathering veterans' symptoms under the umbrella of moral injuries. While PTSD Criterion A requires identification of an event that threatened one's physical survival, Nash and Britt extend the conceptual reach of the threat to moral and spiritual assaults on the person. They claim that service members may develop PTSD symptoms in response to "war-zone events that inflict damage to moral belief systems rather than threats to personal life and safety" (p. 366). They also stress the role of guilt, shame, and self-blame as symptoms of moral injury. Indeed, the Marine Corps includes the category in its Combat and Operational Stress Control manual: "stress arising due to moral damage from carrying out or bearing witness to acts or failures to act that violate deeply held belief systems" (United States Marine Corps, 2010). Some Marines find the concept of moral injury insulting, however, in that the term may reinforce cultural stereotypes of combat veterans as prone to moral lapses (McClosky, 2011).

During a training exercise at Joint Base Lewis–McChord for the 113th Medical Detachment, the unit I was following to Afghanistan, the Army Sergeant overseeing the training shared with me his thoughts on mental breakdowns on the battlefield. A 38-year-old infantryman who had served many tours of duty, he acknowledged how war fighting could impair judgment. "You are not going to find people who hate war more than us in the infantry," he explained—something I had heard from other soldiers as well. "You have to be able to keep your moral compass or you couldn't function," he added. The Sergeant went on to describe a harrowing scene in Iraq where several soldiers killed civilians in the area of their post after having lost everything in a massive assault by insurgents. But "the bottom line of it is that every soldier in that company dealt with the same stress and the same conditions," he insisted, "but the rest of the soldiers in that company did the right things." While moral injury encompasses a wide range of crisis situations, at bottom it signifies some loss of faith in the mission, the military command, or the reliability of one's comrades. As the military worked to manage the growing morale problem during the long wars, I wondered if moral injury operated as one more strategy of institutional containment—as just one more cost of warfare that was now factored into military planning.

The concept of moral injury holds some appeal in the professions because it both acknowledges the deep impacts of warfare and introduces a reassuring framework for managing it. Just as trauma doctors are dominant figures on the front lines, those equipped to treat moral injuries join the ranks of those treating the mental casualties of warfare. And, much like physical injuries, the morally injured soldier is brought into the welcoming arms of various rehabilitative programs ("The Shay Moral Injury Center," n.d.).

Clinicians may themselves slide into personality disorder territory as participants in the war machine. There are many institutional settings, from prisons, courts, schools, and workplace settings to military bases, where interactions between professionals and clients take on the quality of a *folie à deux*, a jointly produced pathological state. In his history of psychiatry, Michel Foucault (2013) argues that systems of scientific rationalization underlie modern institutional forms of power. The role of the American Psychological Association in supporting psychologists involved in torture practices, for example, split the organization during the mid-2000s, with close to half of members leaving the APA (Greene, 2016). The controversy centered on the extent of involvement of APA psychologists in developing interrogation techniques widely recognized internationally as forms of torture (Olson, Soldz, & Davis, 2008; Soldz, 2008, 2010, 2011). Initial inquiries by the American Psychological Association (APA) downplayed the role of psychologists, casting them more as observers than interrogators and as acting to prevent abuses of detainees. Critics countered that the presence of psychologists legitimized torture and reinforced the Department of Defense fiction that it could be carried out properly and humanely. Psychoanalysts played leading roles in exposing the complicity of the APA in these practices, including how their involvement went far beyond their professed position as scientific observers (Soldz, 2008, 2010, 2011).

There are many situations where clinicians do operate in zones of ethical ambiguity—where there truly are conflicting pressures not easily reconciled. Many clinicians enter the military to help soldiers and to buffer the destructive toll of warfare. Jim Sardo, an Army Major and psychologist, describes the history of military recruitment of clinicians during World War I and II and how this recruitment drew deeply on the civilian sector. Unlike career military doctors, those mental health professionals serving as reservists were less apt to think of their jobs as "simply getting people back to combat" (personal communication, May 15, 2011). After treating soldiers in war zones and the VA for decades, Raymond Scurfield (2006) poses the question that came to haunt him:

> Is it really in the long-term mental health of those who are suffering combat stress reactions to be stabilized, reinvigorated and returned to duty versus being medically evacuated out of country? It should be of great concern to all of us that in spite of the dearth of empirical data, this premise is completely accepted and promulgated by military mental health officials.
>
> (p. 55)

As Stanley Milgram (1963, 1965) established in his obedience studies, rationalization and displacement of responsibility onto an external authority operate as common ego defenses. Doctors administering lethal shock to soldiers in order to get them on their feet and back to the front during World War I were responding to the intense pressures of the military mission and the command structure. Clinicians in combat stress control units face similar pressures, as do countless other professionals whose job it is to keep people functioning in dysfunctional places.

## Complex PTSD

Posttraumatic stress disorder draws on conventional storytelling practices in its reliance on a simple narrative structure: The disturbance has a beginning, a middle, and an end. The "post" element of PTSD is based on the idea that a life-threatening situation in the past is experienced *as though it were still present*. Yet for vast numbers of people, the origins of their suffering and harms endured reach far back in time and extend into the foreseeable future. There is no readily accessible site of post-trauma, no language to locate the complaints within the bounds of DSM treatable conditions. In her path-breaking book, *Trauma and Recovery*, Judith Herman (1992) takes up the cause of women diagnosed as borderline personality disorder as well as other conditions she argues are caused by childhood sexual trauma. She places the accounts of sexual survivors within the political landscape of the atrocities of war and the Holocaust, as well as within the smaller-scale tragic dramas of inner-city violence and domestic battering. A common feature, according to Hermann, is the inevitable tension between the "will to deny horrible events and the will to proclaim them aloud" (p. 7). Yet this characterization may say more about the tensions and battles among experts themselves than it does about states of tension in victims. As the "will to deny horrible events" came to be understood as a feature of PTSD, experts stepped in to do much of the proclaiming.

Along with other trauma theorists working in the field of childhood sexual abuse, Herman (1992) led the fight to expand PTSD to include complex trauma. As she assesses the problem, "the existing diagnostic criteria for this disorder are derived mainly from survivors of circumscribed traumatic events. They are based on the prototypes of combat, disaster, and rape" (p. 119). Herman includes under the rubric of complex PTSD clusters of symptoms historically associated with personality disorders, from disturbances in relating to others and affect and mood dysregulation, to antisocial behavior. Hermann joined forces with other socially conscious clinicians to bear witness to suffering beyond the diagnostic terrain of PTSD in calling for official recognition of complex PTSD—a condition associated with long-term exposure to severe forms of abuse and/or neglect.

Overburdened by the expansion of PTSD in the 1990s and 2000s, the DSM Committee has repeatedly balked at extending the category further. As Spitzer, First, and Wakefield (2007) explain in thinly veiled frustration: "Since its introduction into DSM-III in 1980, no other DSM diagnosis, with the exception of Dissociative Identity Disorder (a related disorder), has generated so much controversy in the field" (p. 233).

Boundary-setting efforts to tighten PTSD operate as a professional defense against recognizing the complexity of mental disorders, and particularly this category that explicitly acknowledges pathogenic societal causes. In response to calls for broadening PTSD, the DSM Committee imposes linguistic control with obsessive vigor. Indeed, the description of changes registers the level of anxiety associated with bringing the diagnosis under control. In summarizing DSM-5 changes to criterion A, Weathers, Marx, Friedman, and Schunner (2014) describe the DSM tightening strategy:

> Experiencing and witnessing (a traumatic event) were both retained, although somewhat more emphatically as "directly experiencing" and "witnessing, in person." In addition, two forms of indirect exposure were included. One is the ambiguous "confronted with" from DSM-IV, which was replaced with "learning that the traumatic event(s) occurred to a close family member or close friend." Importantly, this form of indirect exposure was substantially restricted by a new requirement that events involving the actual or threatened death of a loved one must have been violent or accidental.
>
> (p. 97)

Although many clinicians accept the validity of the concept of complex PTSD (Leonard, 2018), the diagnosis has failed to secure official recognition. The migration of PTSD from street psychiatry to official insider is particularly instructive as an illustration of a boundary crisis in the mental health professions. In order to secure passage for new diagnoses into the DSM, proponents must demonstrate that the condition differs from the normal range of suffering to which humans are subjected. In diagnosing an entire region of the world or social class of sufferers as victims of PTSD, the job of mental health workers could be exhaustingly boundless.

The differential diagnosis of PTSD—rules of inclusion and exclusion—can be as murky as distinguishing cultures along national borders carved out by far-away rulers. In everyday life, the differences might not matter. But with a great deal at stake in distributing resources, even small distinctions can assume enormous significance. With law-and-order campaigns shaping how psychiatry rationalized treatment during the 1980s and 1990s, the personality disorders were excluded as pleas, such as the insanity defense, that were the basis of admission to state psychiatric hospitals. A diagnosis of personality disorder routinely cast the defendant's fate within the prison system, even though childhood trauma and severe abuse are highly associated with both criminality and the development of personality disorders.

The fight for acceptance of PTSD into the DSM meant leaving many socially produced traumas behind, in part because the diagnosis bound the condition to something that happened in the past and established the reaction as "post." Further, the focus on identifying an event "outside the range of everyday experience" excluded much of the routine experiences of people subjected to police state repression or chronic poverty. One could argue that PTSD was caused by a natural disaster, such as floods or hurricanes, or human causes, such as combat, rape, or incest. But bringing poverty, urban violence, and the insults and abuses of marginalized groups into the PTSD psychiatric fold indicted the entire social welfare system and structures of inequality. The betrayal of poor Black communities during and after Hurricane Katrina serves as one such example of a collective trauma that failed to generate the same psychiatric outcry as did the mental breakdown of soldiers.

## Warfare and Gender Maladies

One of the post-war anxieties often marginalized by the battlefield horrors of combat veterans' centers on uneasiness over how warfare effects codes of masculinity. From World War I through the Korean War, emotionally broken soldiers, whether described as shell-shocked or battle fatigued, were cast in the psychiatric literature in passive poses—as socially castrated (Showalter, 1985). Ronald Fairbairn (1943) interpreted war neurosis as a symptom of the soldier's unresolved infantile dependencies. Although the "post-Vietnam syndrome" was often portrayed as an effect of America's impotence in the face of its first defeat in a major war, the angry Vietnam veteran entered into the lexicon as a feature of the Vietnam syndrome (Shatan, 1972). Each major war has produced its own version of a masculinity crisis centered on veterans' reactions to a changing post-war cultural landscape (Roper, 2005; Shay, 2003; Whitworth, 2008).

Feminists enlisted the combat narrative of trauma during the 1970s and 1980s in documenting parallels between survivors of war and survivors of rape and domestic abuse (Herman, 1992). The legitimacy of trauma stories has tended to require a moral banner of heroic proportions. There are no morally conflicted, irrational women in the plots of the female trauma survivors described by Judith Herman (1992)—an understandable corrective to the legacy of women-blaming. "Women learn that in rape they are not only violated but dishonored," Herman suggests, and that they suffer "greater contempt than defeated soldiers" (p. 39). This positioning of female survivors of sexual abuse demanded the same dignity that soldiers summon through combat.

Herman (1992) also brought the moral position of the bystander into therapeutic discourses: "Those who bear witness are caught between victim and perpetrator. It is morally impossible to remain neutral in this conflict. The bystander is forced to take sides" (p. 46). Once positions were staked within the either/or political framework of victim and perpetrator, however, it became difficult to challenge the stories that constituted those categories, particularly those associated with the victim position. Yet, people may be both victim and perpetrator, depending on the context and shifting terrain of the conflict. When Herman is describing posttraumatic stress disorder among Vietnam veterans, she is on the side of male victims of war. When she is describing these same damaged men in the context of domestic violence, these male victims assume the role of archetypal perpetrator. And in its focus on absolute moral categories, the trauma model tends to repress the complexity of victim/perpetrator dynamics. The myriad conservative uses of victim politics, for example, the use of "victims' rights" in calls for increased criminal penalties, are obscured in the righteous fervor of many feminist campaigns (Haaken, 2010).

One of the problematic tendencies of the trauma recovery movement is its reliance on extreme cases to stand for a wider continuum of disturbing experiences. Drawing on Amnesty International's chart of coercion for torture victims, Judith Herman (1992) notes that these same techniques are used to subjugate women, in prostitution, in pornography, and in the home. Much like prisoners of war, survivors of domestic violence and sexual abuse describe their loss of personal privacy, how their husbands, fathers, or boyfriends control and regulate their movements and contacts with the outside world. Herman also points out how perpetrators of domestic violence seek to destroy the woman's sense of autonomy by depriving her of food, sleep, or exercise. Victims of various forms of violence may come to identify with the aggressor, who is the precarious link in what remains of the social chain of survival. "Once the perpetrator has succeeded in establishing day-to-day bodily control of the victim," Herman adds, "he becomes a source not only of fear and humiliation but also of solace" (p. 78).

The positions of victim and perpetrator are dynamically related, as the literature on "cycles of violence" has long claimed. Victimized children sometimes grow up to victimize their own children; soldiers sometimes return home and continue the war on the domestic front. But the question of whether traumatic experiences are "re-enacted" later in life depends on many factors. Herman may be suggesting that in any particular contest between a victim and a perpetrator, one must take the side of the less powerful person, the victim, over against the more powerful perpetrator. We may grant some credence to this stance—as a general principle or orienting value—while still recognizing the pitfalls in absolving or condemning individuals based on whether they are placed in one or the other category. At the same time, we may recognize situations where lines need to be decisively drawn between the guilty and the innocent, the oppressor and the oppressed. Herman (1992) does force us to consider commonalities in victimization experiences, from concentration camp survivor and war veteran to victims of rape and sexual assault. But this widening of the lens is accompanied by a costly loss of specificity in the nature of experiences that give rise to trauma claims and how claims are made visible within a moral arena of responsibility.

## Conclusions

Posttraumatic stress disorder represented a revolt against psychiatric hegemony, even as proponents fought for recognition from this same hegemonic enterprise of the American Psychiatric Association. Cautioning that normal people were routinely misdiagnosed as mentally ill or personality disordered, PTSD advocates created more humanized clinical portraits of victims of various abuses. But this strategy created a double-bind. Normalcy relied on categories of the abnormal in crossing the perilous threshold from redeemable to less redeemable conditions.

Reliance on normalcy in summoning public sympathies for disturbed individuals inadvertently reproduces a societal form of splitting. The diagnosis provides a defense for clinicians in managing the contradictory pressures that are most palpable in military and criminal justice settings. PTSD emerged as a strategy for telling stories about why some people come to be seen as antisocial or sociopathic. But this splitting between the good and bad diagnoses separated off from the social field of psychiatry a deeper and more troubling problem: What about people who have been damaged in life in ways that don't conform to the PTSD diagnostic narrative?

The personality disorders have long been recognized as the least reliable diagnoses—a finding that is not merely an artifact of inadequate research studies. The diagnoses are unreliable because clinicians are often aware of how consequential they are for the fates of people caught in the punitive and dehumanizing criminal justice system. Although some researchers note that institutions often produce the very personality effects that are associated with personality disorders, this problem is deeply downplayed in the field of psychiatry. The "ghosts of the sociopath" continue to haunt psychiatry because the field has not as a whole come to terms with its guilty conscience. These ghosts will continue to haunt the field until the profession comes to terms with the extent to which the most damning of the diagnoses continue to be used to discard vast numbers of people as damaged beyond repair.

The next chapter follows a pathway that brought PTSD center stage in psychiatric discourse because it meets at the intersection between psychiatry and biological medicine. The idea that the body tells a story of trauma took hold in trauma theory, making use of a psychoanalytic heuristic that dates back to Freud: the idea that the symptom tells a story. Whereas experts in the criminal justice system and military proceedings enlist PTSD to separate the virtuous from the villainous, the innocent and the damned, the next chapter follows the migrations of the diagnosis in settings where experts read medical signs to separate the physically sick from the mentally ill.

## References

Alford, C. F. (2009). *The Holocaust is not traumatic: The Holocaust can be represented*. Presented at the Annual Meeting of the Political Science Association, Toronto, Canada.

Alford, C. F. (2018). Trauma and psychoanalysis: Freud, Bion, and Mitchell. *Psychoanalysis, Culture & Society, 23*(1), 43–53. https://doi.org/10.1057/s41282-018-0070-7

American Law Institute. *Model Penal Code*. 4.01 § (1961).

American Psychiatric Association. (2013). *Diagnostic and statistical manual of mental disorders (DSM-5)*. Washington, DC: Author.

Anderson, J. (1972, May 23). Calley could have "copped out." *Sarasota Herald-Tribune*, p. 8A. Retrieved from https://news.google.com/newspapers?id=UroqAAAAIBAJ& sjid=kmYEAAAAIBAJ&dq=insanity+plea+military-court&pg=7355,2976455& hl=en

Archer, D., & Gartner, R. (1992). Peacetime casualties: The effects of war on the violent behavior of noncombatants. In E. Aronson (Ed.), *Readings about the social animal* (6th ed., pp. 327–338). New York, NY: W. H. Freeman and Company.

Bonn, S. (2016, October 23). *Diagnosing psychopaths* [Web log post]. Retrieved December 8, 2019, from Psychology Today website: www.psychologytoday.com/ blog/wicked-deeds/201610/diagnosing-psychopaths

Borgida, E., & White, P. (1978). Social perception of rape victims: The impact of legal reform. *Law and Human Behavior, 2*(4), 339–351. https://doi.org/10.1007/ BF01038986

Bremner, J. D., & Marmar, C. R. (2002). *Trauma, memory, and dissociation*. Washington, DC: American Psychiatric Association Publishing.

Brewin, C. R., Andrews, B., & Valentine, J. D. (2000). Meta-analysis of risk factors for posttraumatic stress disorder in trauma-exposed adults. *Journal of Consulting and Clinical Psychology, 68*(5), 748–766. https://doi.org/10.1037/0022-006X.68.5.748

Brunner, J. (2000). Will, desire and experience: Etiology and ideology in the German and Austrian medical discourse on war neuroses, 1914–1922. *Transcultural Psychiatry, 37*(3), 295–320. https://doi.org/10.1177/136346150003700302

Camp, N. M. (2015). *US Army psychiatry in the Vietnam War: New challenges in extended counterinsurgency warfare*. Washington, DC: Government Printing Office.

Cavenar, J. O., & Nash, J. L. (1976). The effects of combat on the normal personality: War neurosis in Vietnam returnees. *Comprehensive Psychiatry*, *17*(5), 647–653. https://doi.org/10.1016/S0010-440X(76)80009-0

Culp, R., Youstin, T. J., Englander, K., & Lynch, J. (2013). From war to prison: Examining the relationship between military service and criminal activity. *Justice Quarterly*, *30*(4), 651–680. https://doi.org/10.1080/07418825.2011.615755

Dean, J. C., & Poremba, G. A. (1983). The alcoholic stigma and the disease concept. *International Journal of the Addictions*, *18*(5), 739–751. https://doi.org/10.3109/10826088309027366

Drescher, J. (2015). Out of DSM: Depathologizing homosexuality. *Behavioral Sciences*, *5*(4), 565–575. https://doi.org/10.3390/bs5040565

Dunnaback, J. (2015). Command responsibility: A small-unit leader's perspective. *Northwestern University Law Review*, *108*(4), 1385–1422. Retrieved from https://scholarlycommons.law.northwestern.edu/nulr/vol108/iss4/6

Effect of qualifying mental disorder guilty except for insanity. 16 2017 Oregon Revised Statutes § 161.295 (2017).

Elbogen, E. B., Johnson, S. C., Newton, V. M., Straits-Troster, K., Vasterling, J. J., Wagner, H. R., & Beckham, J. C. (2012). Criminal justice involvement, trauma, and negative affect in Iraq and Afghanistan war era veterans. *Journal of Consulting and Clinical Psychology*, *80*(6), 1097–1102. https://doi.org/10.1037/a0029967

Fairbairn, W. R. D. (1943). The war neuroses: Their nature and significance. *The British Medical Journal*, *1*(4284), 183–186. Retrieved from www.jstor.org/stable/20325356

Foucault, M. (1975). *Discipline and punish: The birth of the prison* (A. Sheridan, Trans.). New York, NY: Pantheon Books.

Foucault, M. (2013). *History of madness* (J. Khalfa, Ed. and J. Murphy, Trans.). New York, NY: Routledge.

Frequently Asked Questions about Moral Injury. (n.d.). Retrieved December 19, 2019, from The Shay Moral Injury Center at Volunteers of America website: www.voa.org/moral-injury-center/moral-injury-faqs

Freud, S. (1921). Introduction. In Ernest Jones (Ed.), *Psycho-analysis and the war neuroses* (pp. 1–5). London, UK: The International Psycho-Analytical Press.

Freud, S. (1924, 1959). *The standard edition of the complete psychological works of Sigmund Freud volume XX (1925–1926): An autobiographical study, inhibitions, symptoms and anxiety, lay analysis, and other works* (J. Strachey, Ed.). London, UK: The Hogarth Press.

Goffman, E. (1961). *Asylums: Essays on the social situation of mental patients and other inmates*. New York, NY: Penguin Random House.

Greene, S. (2016, August 4). Do no harm: The American Psychological Association wavers on its detainee policy. *The Colorado Independent*. Retrieved from www.coloradoindependent.com/160550/do-no-harm-apa-enhanced-interrogation-ethics-denver

Haaken, J. (1998). *Pillar of salt: Gender, memory, and the perils of looking back*. New Brunswick, NJ: Rutgers University Press.

Haaken, J. (2010). *Hard knocks: Domestic violence and the psychology of storytelling*. New York, NY: Routledge.

Haaken, J. (2013). *Guilty except for insanity: Maddening journeys through an American asylum* [Documentary]. Retrieved from www.guiltyexcept.com/sponsors

Haaken, J. (2017). Many mornings after: Campus sexual assault and feminist politics. *Family Relations, 66*(1), 17–28. https://doi.org/10.1111/fare.12227

Herman, J. L. (1992). *Trauma and recovery: The aftermath of violence—From domestic abuse to political terror* (Rev. ed.). New York, NY: Basic Books.

Hyams, K. C., & Wignall, F. S. (1996). War syndrome and their evaluation: From the U.S. Civil War to the Persian Gulf War. *Annals of Internal Medicine, 125*(5), 398–405.

Jones, E., & Wessely, S. (2007). A paradigm shift in the conceptualization of psychological trauma in the 20th century. *Journal of Anxiety Disorders, 21*(2), 164–175. https://doi.org/10.1016/j.janxdis.2006.09.009

Kloocke, R., Schmiedebach, H.-P., & Priebe, S. (2005). Psychological injury in the two World Wars: Changing concepts and terms in German psychiatry. *History of Psychiatry, 16*(1), 43–60. https://doi.org/10.1177/0957154X05044600

Lawrence, Q. (2015, December 7). *Defying stereotypes, number of incarcerated veterans In U.S. drops* [Audio podcast]. Retrieved December 8, 2019, from www. npr.org/sections/thetwo-way/2015/12/07/458501774/defying-stereotypes-number-of-incarcerated-veterans-in-u-s-drops

Leonard, J. (2018, August 28). *Complex PTSD: Symptoms, behaviors, and recovery* [News]. Retrieved from Medical News Today website: www.medicalnewstoday.com/articles/322886.php

Leroux, T. C. (2015). U.S. military discharges and pre-existing personality disorders: A health policy review. *Administration and Policy in Mental Health and Mental Health Services Research, 42*(6), 748–755. https://doi.org/10.1007/s10488-014-0611-z

Leys, R. (2000). *Trauma: A genealogy.* Chicago, IL: University of Chicago Press.

Lifton, R. J. (1980). On the consciousness of holocaust. *Psychohistory Review, 9*(1), 3–22.

Lifton, R. J. (1985). *Home from the war: Vietnam veterans: Neither victims nor executioners.* New York, NY: Basic Books.

Lynam, D. R., & Vachon, D. D. (2012). Antisocial personality disorder in DSM-5: Missteps and missed opportunities. *Personality Disorders: Theory, Research, and Treatment, 3*(4), 483–495. https://doi.org/10.1037/per0000006

McClosky, M. (2011, April 28). Combat stress as "moral injury" offends Marines. *Stars and Stripes.* Retrieved from www.stripes.com/blogs/stripes-central/stripes-central-1.8040/combat-stress-as-moral-injury-offends-marines-1.142177

McCormick-Goodhart, M. A. (2012). Leaving no veteran behind: Policies and perspectives on combat trauma, veterans courts, and the rehabilitative approach to criminal behavior. *Penn State Law Review, 117*(3), 895–926.

McNally, R. J. (2003). Progress and controversy in the study of posttraumatic stress disorder. *Annual Review of Psychology, 54*, 229–252. https://doi.org/10.1146/annurev.psych.54.101601.145112

Mellsop, G., Varghese, F., Joshua, S., & Hicks, A. (1982). The reliability of Axis II of DSM-III. *American Journal of Psychiatry, 139*(10), 1360–1361. https://doi.org/10.1176/ajp.139.10.1360

Menninger, W. C. (1948). *Psychiatry in a troubled world: Yesterday's war and today's challenge.* Oxford, England: Macmillan Publishers.

Milgram, S. (1963). Behavioral study of obedience. *The Journal of Abnormal and Social Psychology, 67*(4), 371–378.

Milgram, S. (1965). Liberating effects of group pressure. *Journal of Personality and Social Psychology*, *1*(2), 127–134. https://doi.org/10.1037/h0021650

Miller, H. C., & Miller, E. (1940). *The neuroses in war*. London, UK: Macmillan Publishers.

Nash, W. P., & Litz, B. T. (2013). Moral injury: A mechanism for war-related psychological trauma in military family members. *Clinical Child and Family Psychology Review*, *16*(4), 365–375.

Olson, B., Soldz, S., & Davis, M. (2008). The ethics of interrogation and the American Psychological Association: A critique of policy and process. *Philosophy, Ethics, and Humanities in Medicine*, *3*(3). https://doi.org/10.1186/1747-5341-3-3

Pickersgill, M. (2012). Standardising antisocial personality disorder: The social shaping of a psychiatric technology. *Sociology of Health & Illness*, *34*(4), 544–559. https://doi.org/10.1111/j.1467-9566.2011.01404.x

Prot, K. (2010). Research on consequences of the Holocaust. *Archives of Psychiatry and Psychotherapy*, *2*, 61–69.

Roberts-Pedersen, E. (2012). A weak spot in the personality? Conceptualising "war neurosis" in British medical literature of the Second World War. *Australian Journal of Politics and History*, *58*(3), 408–420.

Rogers, R. (2003). Standardizing DSM-IV diagnoses: The clinical applications of structured interviews. *Journal of Personality Assessment*, *81*(3), 220–225. https://doi.org/10.1207/S15327752JPA8103_04

Roper, M. (2005). Between manliness and masculinity: The "war generation" and the psychology of fear in Britain, 1914–1950. *Journal of British Studies*, *44*(2), 343–362. https://doi.org/10.1086/427130

Russell, M. C., Schaubel, S. R., & Figley, C. R. (2018). The darker side of military mental healthcare part two: Five harmful strategies to manage its mental health dilemma. *Psychological Injury and Law*, *11*(1), 37–68. https://doi.org/10.1007/s12207-017-9311-9

Scott, W. J. (1990). PTSD in DSM-III: A case in the politics of diagnosis and disease. *Social Problems*, *37*(3), 294–310.

Scurfield, R. M. (2006). *War trauma: Lessons unlearned, from Vietnam to Iraq*. New York, NY: Algora Publishing.

Shatan, C. F. (1972, May 6). Post-Vietnam syndrome. *The New York Times*. Retrieved from www.nytimes.com/1972/05/06/archives/postvietnam-syndrome.html

Shay, J. (1994). *Achilles in Vietnam: Combat trauma and the undoing of character*. New York, NY: Simon and Schuster.

Shay, J. (2003). *Odysseus in America: Combat trauma and the trials of homecoming*. New York, NY: Simon and Schuster.

Shein, M. G. (2010, September). Post-traumatic stress disorder in the criminal justice system: From Vietnam to Iraq and Afghanistan. *The Federal Lawyer*, 42–49.

Shephard, B. (2003). *A war of nerves: Soldiers and psychiatrists in the twentieth century*. Cambridge, MA: Harvard University Press.

Showalter, E. (1985). *The female malady: Women, madness, and English culture, 1830–1980*. London, UK: Penguin Random House.

Slattery, M., Dugger, M. T., Lamb, T. A., & Williams, L. (2013). Catch, treat, and release: Veteran treatment courts address the challenges of returning home. *Substance Use & Misuse*, *48*(10), 922–932. https://doi.org/10.3109/10826084.2013.797468

Smith, G. E., & Pear, T. H. (1917). *Shell shock and its lessons*. Manchester, England: Manchester University Press.

Soldz, S. (2008). Healers or interrogators: Psychology and the United States torture regime. *Psychoanalytic Dialogues, 18*(5), 592–613. https://doi.org/10.1080/10481880802297624

Soldz, S. (2010). Psychologists defying torture. In A. Harris & S. Botticelli (Eds.), *First do no harm: The paradoxical encounters of psychoanalysis, warmaking, and resistance* (pp. 67–105). New York, NY: Routledge.

Soldz, S. (2011). Fighting torture and psychologist complicity. *Peace Review, 23*(1), 12–20. https://doi.org/10.1080/10402659.2011.548240

Spitzer, C., Barnow, S., Völzke, H., John, U., Freyberger, H. J., & Grabe, H. J. (2009). Trauma, posttraumatic stress disorder, and physical illness: Findings from the general population. *Psychosomatic Medicine, 71*(9), 1012–1017. https://doi.org/10.1097/PSY.0b013e3181bc76b5

Spitzer, R. L., First, M. B., & Wakefield, J. C. (2007). Saving PTSD from itself in DSM-V. *Journal of Anxiety Disorders, 21*(2), 233–241. Retrieved from www.beforeyoutakethatpill.com/2009/3/spitzer.pdf

Stone, A. A. (1993). Post-traumatic stress disorder and the law: Critical review of the new frontier. *Journal of the American Academy of Psychiatry and the Law Online, 21*(1), 23–36. Retrieved from www.jaapl.org/content/21/1/23

Trestman, R. L. (2014). DSM-5 and personality disorders: Where did Axis II go? [Special section]. *The Journal of the American Academy of Psychiatry and the Law, 42*(2), 141–145.

Trull, T. J. (2011). Challenges in the study of personality and psychopathology. *World Psychiatry, 10*(2), 113–115. Retrieved from www.ncbi.nlm.nih.gov/pmc/articles/PMC3104885/

United States Marine Corps. (2010, December). *Combat and operational stress control*. Retrieved from www.marines.mil/Portals/59/Publications/MCTP%203-30E%20Formerly%20MCRP%206-11C.pdf?ver=2017-09-28-081327-517

Van der Kolk, B. A. (2000). Trauma, neuroscience, and the etiology of hysteria: An exploration of the relevance of Breuer and Freud's 1893 article in light of modern science. *Journal of the American Academy of Psychoanalysis, 28*(2), 237–262.

Vaughan, B. (2015, October 21). Robert Bales speaks: Confessions of America's most notorious war criminal. *GQ*. Retrieved from www.gq.com/story/robert-bales-interview-afghanistan-massacre

Walls, S. (2010). The need for special veteran courts. *Denver Journal of International Law and Policy, 39*, 695–729. Retrieved from http://heinonline.org/HOL/Page?handle=hein.journals/denilp39&id=717&div=&collection=

Wead, S. (2015). Ethics, combat, and a soldier's decision to kill. *Military Review*, 69–81. Retrieved from www.armyupress.army.mil/Portals/7/military-review/Archives/English/MilitaryReview_20150430_art013.pdf

Weathers, F. W., Marx, B. P., Friedman, M. J., & Schnurr, P. P. (2014). Posttraumatic stress disorder in DSM-5: New criteria, new measures, and implications for assessment. *Psychological Injury and Law, 7*(2), 93–107.

Whitworth, S. (2008). Militarized masculinity and post-traumatic stress disorder. In J. L. Parpart & M. Zalewski (Eds.), *Rethinking the man question: Sex, gender and violence in international relations.* (pp. 109–126). London, UK: Zed Books.

Wilson, J. P. (1994). The historical evolution of PTSD diagnostic criteria: From Freud to DSM-IV. *Journal of Traumatic Stress*, *7*(4), 681–698. https://doi.org/10.1007/BF02103015

Wilson, M. (1993). DSM-III and the transformation of American psychiatry: A history. *American Journal of Psychiatry*, *150*(3), 399–410. https://doi.org/10.1176/ajp.150.3.399

Zaretsky, E. (2005). *Secrets of the soul: A social and cultural history of psychoanalysis.* New York, NY: Vintage.

# Chapter 3

# Psychic Trauma and the Body

During the early 20th century, a wave of disturbing stories captured the news in Germany, igniting controversy in the medical community. Reports of telephone operators seized by inexplicable bolts of shock as they answered calls on their switchboards poured into the accident insurance offices. The typical case involved distressing sensations located in the head, such as numbness and pain, and general fatigue. The symptoms followed what operators reported as a sudden surge of electricity through their headpieces. Historian Andreas Killen (2003) explains how the operators' stories began with the same complaint: "I suffered a shock." When inspectors could find no material explanation for the syndrome, doctors were summoned to review the reports, diagnosing many of the women as suffering from emotional trauma following exposure to a shock to the nervous system. The prevailing medical thinking at the time was that small surges of electrical activity could produce damage to the nervous system—damage that could be difficult to detect. As insurance claims based on the condition mounted, many of these same doctors reversed position in support of a German law in the 1920s to disallow benefits based on the diagnosis. Killen offers that physicians were tone-deaf to the exhaustion of phone operators taking up to 150 calls per hour and collapsing during grueling speed-ups. He presents the case as a cautionary tale on the role of physicians in translating work stress into the dramaturgy of psychic trauma, and of what happens when the drama fails to cross the threshold of recognition within the prevailing medical model. Physicians emerged as arbiters of the complaints of these workers but they operated within a narrow framework of visibility. As Killen explains, "entitlement to benefits was made contingent upon proof of a direct causal connection to an accident, while long-term occupational hazards, such as chronic over-exertion, were expressly exempted from coverage" (p. 206).

This book builds on one of Sigmund Freud's early contributions to the field of psychiatry: the idea that the symptom tells a story. But the meaning of the story depends on professional translators. Rather than the broken machine model of mental disorder, Freud approached the symptom as an unconscious communication. In the case of hysteria, he argued, the patient unconsciously relinquishes control over a part of the body in order to escape an unbearable conflict. If the soldier can't move his arm, he can't lift a weapon to kill the enemy. If an operator can't hear, she can't pick up those calls. This form of hysteria came to be described as a conversion disorder. In the case of the telephone operators, Freudian analysts might recognize signs of group hysteria as the idea of psychic shock and its associated dramaturgy took hold among the exhausted workers. Indeed, the idea that unconscious conflict can be converted into bodily dysfunction continues to be recognized as a hallmark feature of psychosomatic conditions (Ali et al., 2015). Assen Jablensky (1999) explains the common clinical picture of somatic conditions: "they tend to behave (to paraphrase Freud) 'as though anatomy did not exist'" (p. 4).

Psychiatry emerged as a field within medicine to bridge this gap in the communicative logic of symptomatology. Yet, establishing causal links between psychological processes and physical symptomatology remains one of the most vexing problems in psychiatry. Decades of research efforts to link genetic, hormonal, and neurochemical factors to specific mental disorders have made casual links more elusive than ever. In any given disorder, hundreds of causal factors may be implicated, each of which can be implicated in other conditions as well. Although physical diseases may similarly involve a complex and indeterminate set of factors, their scientific validity as medical conditions rely on establishing a primary set of pathogens.

The American Psychiatric Association (2013) sought to bridge the ontological gap between mental and medical disorders in the DSM-5 by defining mental disorders as patterns or syndromes in individuals based on an "underlying psychobiological dysfunction." In characterizing this grounding of psychiatric diagnoses in biological causes, Jeffrey Lacasse (2014) sardonically describes DSM-5 as merely an expensive medical dictionary. Others applaud the APA campaign to tie the fate of the field to biomedical research. Joaquim Raese (2015), for example, laments what he views as the dualism that stubbornly persists as a mode of thinking in psychiatry:

> It is a discipline built on a fault line straddling the tectonic plate of neuroscience, which includes neuro-psychopharmacology and other biological treatments on the one hand, and the tectonic plate of the "psychosocial" which includes a host of psychotherapies and social systems interventions.
>
> (para. 1)

Working at these fault lines means clinging to one tectonic plate or the other, and biological treatments have tended to hold the ground historically over the psychosocial.

In this chapter, I trace the history of an idea that captured trauma therapists in the late 20th century—the idea that psychic trauma presents itself through a medical symptom. The tensions in psychiatry over how mental disturbances are converted into somatic symptoms is an important part of the PTSD story. Although physiological correlates of stress reactions are well established in medical science, indicators of psychic trauma are murkier. All animals have evolved with capacities to react to threats—what are commonly termed fight/flight autonomic responses. Threat perception stimulates the nervous system—increased heart rate and blood pressure, as well as increased adrenal output in the form of adrenaline and cortisol. This constellation of physiological reactions, termed the human stress response, carries survival value in the short run but is associated with serious health problems over the longer term.

In the Introduction to the book, I describe the union of stress research and trauma studies in the PTSD movement and how this union was strained from the start. The concept of posttraumatic stress situated a widening array of psychiatric conditions in the context of a universal and relatively non-controversial area of medicine—the human stress response. Links between stress and trauma were important in the founding of the early PTSD movement, particularly in normalizing disorders that were highly stigmatized. Further, the stress response was established biological science. A key premise of the PTSD diagnosis centered on the idea that some stressors could overwhelm the body's normal stress response, including the mind's ego defenses. Once dynamic mental systems enter the picture, however, along with the historical and cultural determinants of how events are perceived and mentally processed, the human stress response gathers up considerable complexity. Yet this complex web of determinants tends to be dissociated from the trauma models circulating in psychiatry.

Tracing concepts of psychic trauma requires a return here to military medicine and lessons from the battlefield. Trauma medicine has deep roots in the management of battlefield casualties, contexts where mental health providers are routinely enlisted to treat psychiatric casualties. Whereas emergency doctors are trained to intervene in situations involving bodily injury, trauma psychiatry attends to psychic blows that are more elusive. As Jennifer Terry (2017) notes in her history of trauma medicine and warfare, the wars in Afghanistan and Iraq produced enormous advances for trauma care, including in regenerative medicine. Ground troops exposed to IED blasts were more apt to lose limbs than life during these conflicts—war injuries that drove technological advances in artificial limbs and nerve regeneration. While amputees and paraplegics have long been associated with war veterans, Terry describes an element of magical thinking that governs this field and the "technofuturistic hopes that attach to suffering" (p. 86).

For psychiatrists treating psychic trauma, the body remains the privileged location for establishing expertise and for making hidden injuries visible. Psychoanalyst Alice Miller (2006) famously asserted during the 1990s that "the body never lies"—trauma speaks through the body when the mind fails to register its effects. Psychiatrist Bessel van der Kolk (2015) extends this metaphor in *The Body Keeps the Score*, asserting that the effects of psychic trauma are now measurable through standard medical tests. In an interview, van der Kolk explains what he means by keeping score:

> The core issue with trauma is that people feel unsafe in their bodies. . . . The degree to which your body keeps reacting that way defines the depth of your trauma. So, trauma is expressed as sensations of heartbreak, gut wrench, of being irritable, being on edge, or just being numbed out.
>
> (Guzman, 2018)

These same responses are associated with anxiety and stress—responses not in themselves indicators of exposure to trauma. The body may indeed keep the score, but the scoreboard registers competitive strivings among experts as much as it does degrees of mental suffering.

## Boundary Disputes

Presenting complaints in posttraumatic stress disorder often include somatic symptoms (McFarlane, 2017). Health concerns among trauma survivors are not surprising given that stress reactions weaken the body's defenses against illness over time. But two conditions carry the longest history as sites for establishing the medical validity of the concept of psychic trauma: conversion disorder and somatic symptom disorder. Both conditions are listed in the DSM-5 as associated with exposure to trauma. Their histories as diagnoses represent as well sites of crises in the field of psychiatry—crises where concepts of psychic trauma play a leading role.

Scientists increasingly recognize the complex interplay of brain activity and psychophysiological pathways throughout the body. But the specific mechanisms through which mental conflicts or psychic disturbances are expressed through a medical symptom remain highly controversial. Conversion disorder, the taxonomic descendent of hysteria, also termed "functional neurological disorder," is characterized by disturbances in voluntary motor function that cannot be explained medically. Somatic disorder—or somatization disorder—also involves medically unexplained signs and symptoms. But this latter condition involves multiple physical complaints. Whereas conversion reactions are expressed as a dramatic mimicking of a neurological condition, the symptoms associated with somatic disorder tend to be more diffuse and medically vague.

In offering rationales for tightening criteria for the somatic disorders, the border where psychiatry and medical specialties often meet, DSM-5 acknowledges the history of error in assigning psychological etiologies to physical complaints: "The reliability of determining that a somatic symptom is medically unexplained is limited, and grounding a diagnosis on the absence of an explanation is problematic and reinforces mind–body dualism" (American Psychiatric Association, 2013, p. 309). The revised diagnosis under the heading of "somatic symptom disorder" in DSM-5 requires abnormal thoughts as one of the criteria for diagnosis, for example, the elaboration of a delusional system around the physical complaint.

Since the 19th century, psychiatry has produced a range of theories to explain how abnormal mental states manifest through malfunctioning organs—theories inevitably molded through the prejudicial thinking of the time. Many outdated claims, such as phrenological explanations for criminality and the wandering womb theory of hysteria, suffered precipitous collapses in legitimacy. But other mind–body formulations have had more staying power in the professions.

During the 1950s and 1960s, psychoanalytic theories of psychosomatic illness gained currency in psychiatry as part of the larger expansion of psychoanalysis in the field of medicine. Drawing on Freud's insight that zones of the body carried symbolic meaning in psychic development, post-war psychoanalysts such as Franz Alexander (1932; 1950) promoted the idea that physical ailments were caused by unconscious conflict. Asthma sufferers were thought to suffer from suffocating mothers and dependency conflicts, whereas colitis was associated with repressed anger, expressed in the symptom of "angry bowels." Trauma could be part of the clinical picture, but psychosomatic psychiatry relied heavily on Freudian drive theory and concepts of neurosis as effects of blocked energy or inhibitions in the release of intense affects. As Alexander's line of psychoanalytic thinking was discredited in psychiatry in the 1970s, a range of mind–body concepts based on psychogenic etiologies continued to thrive in counter-cultural, non-Western practices during that same era.

The proliferation of somatic treatments in alternative medicine was in no small measure a response to the low status of these conditions in mainstream medicine. Both conversion reactions and somatic disorders are associated with women, rural people, the less educated, and the poor (Ali et al., 2015). Indeed, psychiatry itself emerged as a highly labor-intensive medical specialty and lost status in part because the talking cure scored poorly in American medical metrics established by the technology-driven, profit-oriented specialties. Throughout much of its history of medical recognition, conversion hysteria has been conceptualized as a condition of those less capable of rational thought or less able to control their emotions. Treatment of the nervous conditions of women particularly were conducive to the rise of psychiatry and its early legitimacy. Roy Porter (1993) argues that conversion hysteria spread in the 19th century because of its protean qualities—and its capacity to mimic common medical conditions of interest to physicians. He describes hysteria as a co-constructed condition that allowed forms of distress to be recognized through cultural idioms of illness available to both doctors and their patients, adding that "somaticizing" is not limited to the uneducated. Doctors contribute as well to the somaticizing of mental suffering:

> Affluent New Yorkers are today allowed, even expected, to act out trauma psychologically. Mao's China, by contrast, apparently condemned such performances as lapses into inadmissible subjectivism and political deviancy. Hence "feeling bad" in the Republic had to be couched in terms of a physical debility or malfunction that escaped censure and solicited sympathy and relief.
>
> (p. 228)

Although clinical recognition of emotional distress may no longer require a somatic "host," the process of untangling somatic signs and psychological symptoms routinely eludes the tools of medical experts. The extensive clinical listening involved and the inevitable ambiguities that remain confront the economic mandates of the American health care system as well. As psychiatrist Nada Stotland (2008) points out, "psychosomatic illnesses are thought to consume inordinate amounts of medical attention and are not deemed worthy of that investment" (para. 1). She casts psychosomatic medicine as a field struggling to cast off its pre-scientific roots in psychoanalysis, and she mocks the reasoning of earlier practitioners, "whether to explain wheezing as a cry for one's mother, joint inflammation as a reaction to psychologically unacceptable aggressive impulses, and gastrointestinal ulceration as a reaction to unfulfilled oral strivings" (para. 5).

In rejecting old-school Freudian thinking, Stotland (2008) takes up psychic trauma as the terrain where psychosomatic medicine learns to listen differently to patients' complaints, and particularly to women's complaints. Somatic symptoms often tell a story of past sexual or physical abuse, Stotland suggests, but the story requires a receptive listener. "During the typical doctor–patient interaction, less than 2 minutes elapse from the time the patient begins to explain the reason for her visit to the time she is interrupted by specific, rapid-fire questions from the doctor" (para. 22). From this social psychological perspective, the diagnosis of psychosomatic illness is as much a disorder of the practitioner and the health care system as it is the patient. Her guidelines for practice extend psychosomatic medicine into the psychotherapeutic realm of listening with a third ear. But these stories may be limiting as well, particularly if doctors are primarily attuned to hidden indicators of trauma.

## Palpable Suffering: Nervous Bodies

In the course of interviewing patients at the Oregon State Hospital, I routinely asked about their understandings of their diagnosis and whether it fits with their own thinking about their problems. One patient told me that while she agreed with her diagnosis of acute psychosis, not otherwise specified (NOS), she thought the doctors had overlooked the actual cause of her breakdown. While her chart included a long list of bizarre behaviors focused on putting objects in her anus and a range of creative means of purging, she insisted that these were attempts to expel the menacing cause of her illness: bacteria in her bowel. This was the primary cause of her crime, she insisted, which was attempted murder of her young son. Colonics have been in and out of fashion throughout the history of psychiatry, largely based on this idea that toxins circulating from the bowel can produce pathological mental states. Yet she found little support among her doctors for this age-old etiology of madness. As microbiology comes onto the psychiatric stage of medicine, however, particularly in linking microbes in the gut to brain chemistry, this bowel theory may yet prove to hold as much validity as any other explanation (Cryan & Dinan, 2012; Mayer, Knight, Mazmanian, Cryan, & Tillisch, 2014).

Throughout the 19th century, mental suffering secured recognition in medicine through the distressed organs that alerted doctors to connections between emotions and illness. During the US Civil War, Jacob Mendes Da Costa, a Caribbean physician and surgeon, treated large numbers of Union soldiers at an Army hospital in Philadelphia. During this same period, physicians were under intense pressure to identify malingering or faking symptoms—a problem thought to be widespread on both the Union and Confederate sides. In 1863, the government issued a requirement that claims of injury be evaluated under ether to determine if the soldier was faking the condition (Connor, 2006). As soldiers were being admitted to his Army hospital for various medical complaints, Da Costa noticed a mysterious pattern. On examination, he found that most of these patients exhibited no physical signs of disease or disorder, even though they complained of symptoms suggestive of heart disease. Later named the *Da Costa syndrome*, the condition included a cluster of circulatory and respiratory ailments. Da Costa concluded from his analysis of 200 cases that 38.5 percent had been exposed to "hard field service and excessive marching" (Meagher, 1919, as cited in National Research Council et al., 2007). Da Costa established what would become a longstanding cornerstone of medical authority—a means of separating the fakers and weak-willed from the truly ill.

Although the Da Costa syndrome generated a vast taxonomy of terms in 19th-century medical literature, from neurocirculatory asthenia, cardiac neurosis, chronic asthenia, effort syndrome, functional cardiovascular disease, to subacute asthenia, the term that captured the popular imagination was the more poetic idiom of *soldier's heart* (Gilbert, 1983; Kinzie & Goetz, 1996; Mackenzie, 1920). The history of psychiatry honors Da Costa for a groundbreaking discovery, but the millions who mourned the dead, those heartbroken families who lost their sons, most certainly found affinity with a term that kept the subject—the soldier—at the center of the condition ascribed to their suffering. The heart carried both symbolic significance as the center of emotional life and foregrounded the concrete visceral life-blood of the fighter.

Da Costa recognized that mental states could lead to symptoms mimicking a physical disease, unwittingly marking a starting point in well over a century of turf wars between doctors of the mind and doctors of the body, with their competing inferences on the causes of patients' complaints. Da Costa's diagnosis bore remarkable similarity to a competing syndrome noted among soldiers for centuries that also involved feeling sick at heart—*nostalgia*. Initially documented by a 17th-century medical student in treating Swiss mercenaries, the illness included intrusive memories, irregular heartbeat, fainting, and anorexia (Roth, 1991). The problem of homesickness—among the most pervasive sources of distress among soldiers and displaced people—required a medical category in order to secure recognition by the state. Both nostalgia and soldier's heart receded in medical and psychiatric discourse by the late 19th century, reduced to footnotes in the trajectory of scientific progress (McCormick-Goodhart, 2012).

Even though symptoms of stress involve hormonal, gastrointestinal, and circulatory systems, neurology became the forerunner of modern psychiatry and its lasting competitor in explaining the mind–brain–body complex. Many of the 19th-century mental maladies, from monomania and hysteria to neurasthenia, were associated with artists and poets as well as women—those thought to be prone to nervous breakdowns. Termed "alienists" in the 19th century, doctors specializing in mental diseases generally worked as superintendents in asylums, treating a loosely categorized assemblage of misfits that shared the condition of *mental alienation* (Shorter, 1997). Modern psychiatry came onto the historical stage through neurology and the treatment of nervous conditions of women, as well as infirmities of "feminine" men (Porter, 1993; Showalter, 1985). Hysteria, derived in etymology from the Greek term for the uterus and from ancient thinking about the pathogenesis of the "wandering womb," served as the prototypical neurosis in the 19th century. While most physicians rejected the idea of a detached womb moving upward in the body to disrupt rational thought, the metaphor fit closely enough with patriarchal medical opinion that the female body was somehow implicated in women's emotional instability.

## Psychic Trauma: The Influence of Jean-Martin Charcot

The French neurologist Jean-Martin Charcot served as midwife to modern psychiatry in making visible the suffering born of psychological trauma. He was able to demonstrate that symptoms of psychic trauma could be produced under hypnosis and established as a distinct functional syndrome with no basis in known neurological pathways. He established, for example, that hysterical paralysis was psychological rather than organic because the pattern of the disability conformed to the subjective contours of the limb rather than to the structure of the nervous system. Through hypnosis, he was also able to elicit the symptoms, primarily as a series of contracted movements culminating in what appeared to be a grand mal seizure. Charcot mapped the symptoms of "epilepto-hysteria" as a series of stages that conformed to standard medical taxonomies for disease. From the back wards of the Salpêtrière hospital in Paris, patients suffering the effects of various social conditions gained recognition in what became the most famous medical stage of the era. The Salpêtrière was the largest hospital in France and one of the largest in the world, housing around 5,000 patients, primarily women. Much like psychiatric hospitals in the Western world today, the Salpêtrière was part prison and part hospital, a place of both confinement and refuge for various misfits, from beggars, epileptics, and syphilitics to prostitutes, religious heretics, and petty thieves (Micale, 1985; Showalter, 1985).

Charcot secured lasting respect for his contributions to the field of neurology, including differential diagnosis of Parkinson's disease and multiple sclerosis (Goetz, 2011). He fell into disrepute late in his career as it was revealed that his assistants were coaching patients in the symptoms Charcot expected in support of his theory of hysteria. Charcot himself produced a rich trove of photographs and documents that add further support to the thesis that the hysterical conditions that mesmerized this physician and his audience of medical observers was in part an artifact of their own fantasies. Lesser known than these dramatic hysterical displays, however, are Charcot's case studies that bring the body into the clinical picture in ways that point to an array of harsh social conditions in the development of hysterical symptoms. Late 19th-century hysteria—as a dramatic performance of disability that mimicked epileptic fits—served defensive functions for physicians such as Charcot who sought to bring diffuse and varying sources of suffering under control.

The era of the 1870s and 1880s, when Charcot rose to prominence as a physician, was a period of fierce competition among mind healers, as each challenged the clergy and religious notions of moral degeneracy. Spiritual mediums inspired a new religious movement in France as well as in other parts of Europe and the United States, enlisting vaguely understood principles of electricity in explaining their ability to communicate at a distance with spirits from the beyond. Mediums, most of whom were women, were hardly in a position to challenge the power of medicine. But they did pose a threat as medical doctors positioned themselves as the dominant authority in the management of nervous conditions.

Charcot (1888) devotes a series of lectures to these competing mind healers, describing hysteria as an epidemic "developed under the influence of the practice of spiritualism" (p. 13). His explanations were no less fanciful, however, than those of the spiritualists. One lecture begins with cases of children of spiritualists, where a mother and father turn to him in desperation to cure their three children of hysterical fits. Charcot identifies hysterical zones on the 13-year-old girl—"stigmata" on her breasts, abdomen, flanks, and calves where touch stimulates a hysterical seizure. Her two younger brothers display more aggressive versions of these seizure-like attacks, Charcot observes, with the least sick of the three suffering sometimes three or four episodes a day. In this case, he identifies the family as the pathogenic influence, ordering separation of the siblings in the institution to limit the contagion effect of contact:

> The whole history of this little family epidemic is, moreover, very instructive. It makes you a witness of the genesis and the evolution of the disease in a family of nervous and arthritic persons. . . . It gives you an idea of the influence exercised by the kind of life one leads and the conditions of habitation. Lastly, it indicates clearly the danger there is, especially to persons nervously predisposed, in superstitious practices.
>
> (p. 12)

Mediums offered dramatic visual displays of their powers during séances, physically embodying the deceased and communicating clairvoyantly with departed loved ones. Mediums served as informal grief counselors, generally offering reassuring messages from the beyond (Haaken, 1998). The rise of spiritualism in late 19th-century Europe and America grew in response to a sustained period of social crisis. By the end of the century, industrial capitalism had transformed the known environment and transported large numbers of people to far-away places, even as experts arose to bridge the distance between the old world and the new.

Professional debates over psychic disturbances and their links to medical pathologies unfolded amid convulsive reactions to the expansion of the railroad system during the 19th century as well. Railway accidents generated a wave of reports of "railway spine," a condition that established Charcot as an authority on psychic trauma. These were cases where victims of train crashes or derailments complained of difficulty standing or walking even though they showed no physical signs of injury. Physicians were summoned to issue their medical opinions, with some taking the position that subtle ruptures to nerves in the spine caused the ailment and others taking the stance that most of the claims were based on faking illness (Erichsen, 1867).

Psychic trauma emerged as a mediating quasi-medical concept. Charcot argued that mental shock could disturb functioning in ways that resemble neurological disorders and that symptoms operate outside of conscious control. He begins with acknowledgment that "the victims of railroad accidents quite naturally claim damages of the companies. The case goes into court; thousands of dollars are at stake" (Charcot, 1888, p. 99). He continues by asserting that many of these cases are "hysteria, nothing but hysteria." Charcot adds that hysteria should not be confused with faking illness or weakness of the will. The task of making such distinctions was burdened by "prejudices profoundly rooted" in the medical profession, Charcot (1888) continues to explain (p. 99). While an "effeminate young man" may succumb to emotional breakdowns, the able-bodied man "may, as the result of a railway accident, a collision, a car running off the track, become hysterical just like a woman" (p. 101). Charcot identifies "terror experienced by the patient at the moment of the accident" as the psychical element of hysteria—a shock to the nervous system that leads to debilitating paralyses and seizure-like fits (p. 115).

One case study in Charcot's lecture series on hysteria prefigures contemporary PTSD narratives in its focus on a traumatic event that produces a delayed set of debilitating symptoms. The young man, "Gui," was a locksmith, 27 years in age and robust in stature. Like most of the cases documented by Charcot, the reported family history includes drunkenness, early death, and many examples of what Charcot (1888) judged to be inherited nervous illness. He reports that the patient, at the age of 12, became extremely fearful and "cowardly, and could not remain alone in a room without a feeling of fear and anxiety" (p. 124). The boy excelled in school, although he developed "an immoderate passion for women and strong drink." At the age of 21, Charcot continues to explain, Gui was attacked by someone with a knife after a night of carousing. As a result, the young man suffered the loss of his left eye.

Charcot (1888) describes symptoms developing about three years later that meet contemporary criteria for PTSD: intrusive imagery, nightmares centered on reliving the attack, intense anxiety, and what Charcot describes as hypnogogic hallucinations. After six months of suffering, the young man "was the victim of a new accident, more terrible than the first" (p. 125). Gui was working on a third-floor balcony when he fell to the street, losing consciousness for about an hour. When he was taken to the hospital, the doctors feared that he had suffered a fracture of his cranium. He recovered and returned home but developed nocturnal hallucinations and terrors, as well as dizziness and trembling. After 18 months of illness, with no remission in his symptoms, Gui was admitted to the Salpêtrière under the care of one of Charcot's associates. The symptoms became more acute, particularly after the patient was transferred to Charcot's ward. Charcot describes Gui as "a man of good muscular development, vigorous," and in generally good health. The patient is mentally alert and socializes well with staff. Charcot then describes in exacting detail the patterns of the shaking and trembling Gui exhibits after being hospitalized on his ward, adding that, "the only hysterogenous zone noted in Gui occupies the testicle and the tract of the spermatic cord almost as far as the groin of the right side" (p. 125). Charcot describes the hysterical attack that is both stimulated and terminated by pressing on a hysterogenous zone, specifically in pinching or compressing the testicles.

Charcot (1888) notes that these attacks conform to those exhibited by the "grand hysteria" of female patients, with the exception of the "clownism"—a distorted facial expression—accompanying the signature arcing movements of the body. "All this part of the seizure is very fine, if I may so express myself, and every one of these details deserves to be fixed by the process of instantaneous photography" (p. 129). This and other cases of male hysteria are described as evidence that hysterical illness can develop in males—a finding bolstering his claim that hysteria is a universal mental disease located in the mind rather than emanating from female reproductive organs.

Through these case histories, Charcot's (1888) clinical portraits provide a window onto the difficult lives of young workers during this era of widespread hardship. Although Charcot's gallery of the hysterics at the Salpêtrière became iconic, his medical travels among the dispossessed have garnered far less historical notice. At the close of the Franco–Prussian War in 1871, with the defeat of France, life in Paris was brutally harsh, including severe food shortages. The Salpêtrière was as much sanctuary for the poor as it was a medical institution. Charcot's case histories provide closely drawn pictures of the lives of many of the working-class people who entered the facility—and the challenges Charcot confronted in identifying predictable medical patterns in their complaints.

Studying at the Salpêtrière in the 1870s, Freud was a great admirer of the "master" while disputing Charcot's focus on heredity. Charcot introduced psychic shock as the proximal cause of hysteria, but he emphasized hereditary factors in creating a vulnerability to the condition. Freud brought memory into the dramaturgy of madness by claiming that the hysteric "suffers from reminiscences." In their chronic state of infirmity, hysterics refused the demands of adult life and remained bound to childhood fears. The body remained the bedrock of medical authority for psychoanalysis as well, however. Freud's close collaborations with Wilhelm Fliess, an ear, nose, and throat specialist, serve as one notorious example. His support for his colleague's "nasal reflex neurosis" theory ended after Fliess's surgical operation on Emma Eckstein as treatment for her depression (Chester, 2007). She came close to death after the botched surgery, bringing the nasal theory of neurosis to an abrupt end. Nonetheless, Freud continued to rely on medical signs, specifically hysterical paralysis, in establishing psychoanalysis as a discipline that occupies an ambiguous border between psychology and medicine.

## Bodies at War

Unlike Da Costa's Civil War soldiers and their heart complaints and general malaise, soldiers during the Great War displayed dramatic symptoms that bore marked similarity to the hysterical symptoms described by Charcot in the 1870s. World War I medical manuals describe "epileptoid" movements as one of the most common conditions among soldiers (Moscovich, Estupinan, Qureshi, & Okun, 2013). These symptoms aroused intense suspicions among military physicians, however, because they could be easily simulated. If Freud was correct in claiming that the symptom tells a story, simulated symptoms also tell a story. While these soldiers likely suffered from many of the same feelings of terror, hyper-vigilance, and helplessness codified under the contemporary category of PTSD, their desire to escape from the lethal power of the war machine confronted severe sanctions. Many soldiers adopted the bodily articulated symptoms of the late 19th-century hysteric, with its dramatic displays of contorted movements. Military doctors enlisted some of the same electrical treatments in use for "weak nerves" to get them back on their feet. The boundary between treatment and torture blurred as pressures on physicians mounted.

Human impulses to retreat from life-threatening situations—indicators of mental health during times of peace—are classified as cowardice or treason in the theater of war. Freud's analysis of shell shock, described in Chapter 2, brought the madness of war closer to home, locating the war neuroses in the command structure of the military rather than solely the result of actions by the enemy. Freud also castigated army doctors for driving soldiers back to the front. Although he had initially supported Germany and the Central Powers, Freud, like major segments of the armed and civilian populations on both sides of the conflict, became increasingly critical of the war effort (Freud, 1921).

Germany was the leading producer of psychiatric knowledge during the Great War and generated a vast encyclopedia of psychiatric terms and typologies. Feelings, thoughts, and impulses that were considered normal in civilian life were, in the context of war, subject to military scrutiny as signs of pathology. Everyday emotional responses entered medical literature in the form of newly discovered syndromes. Reminiscent of the "drapetomania" diagnosis in mid-19th-century America, a condition ascribed to African slaves attempting to escape captivity, psychiatric diagnoses became part of the disciplinary arsenal of the military during World War I. Robert Gaupp, a leading German psychiatrist who introduced the term "fright reaction," was one of those leading military doctors. Common enough among normal soldiers, the reaction was described as an overwhelming wish to flee active duty. Gaupp also describes the more ominous condition of "fright neurosis" that developed among soldiers predisposed to degeneracy or mental instability. Emil Kraepelin, the founder of the earliest classification system in psychiatry, had proposed fright neurosis in place of the broader concept of traumatic neurosis as part of a larger campaign to bring accident claims under control (Crocq & Crocq, 2000). In his autobiography, Kraepelin reflects on the dilemmas for doctors in identifying fakers and malingerers: "This was compounded by the population's feeling of pity for the seemingly severely ill 'war-shakers' [*Kriegszilterer*], who drew attention to themselves on street corners and used to be generously rewarded" (Crocq & Crocq, 2000, para. 23). Hypnosis and suggestive techniques were fortified with more violent methods as war fatigue set in and the task of separating malingerers, war resisters, and battle-weary soldiers became more unwieldy.

Indeed, the diagnosis of war neurosis carried soldiers only so far. In an address to War Congress of the German Psychiatric Association, Gaupp made this principle quite explicit: "Never forget that we physicians have now to put all our work in the service of one mission: to serve our army and our fatherland" (as cited in Shephard, 2003, p. 98). In Germany, particularly, psychiatric discussion of post-war conditions cautioned that chronic mental infirmities, those reactions that persisted after the close of the war or were not responsive to available treatments, were best understood as a form of "pension neurosis"—a political diagnosis taken up in more detail in Chapter 4. Freudian theory and the concept of the unconscious were now enlisted to choreograph a less noble story of the war neurotic; the veteran is now cast as neurotically invested in staying sick and nursing his war injuries.

Throughout the history of psychiatry, researchers and practitioners have repeatedly circled back to a question fraught with political implications—the question of why some people develop symptoms of traumatic neuroses whereas most do not. For those who fail to bounce back from a breakdown, clinical speculations on the causes of their infirmed states are inevitably infused with moral judgments. Psychoanalysis introduced a more complex model of psychic trauma than those offered by other medical specialists—a model of trauma that placed reactions to warfare in the context of childhood fears and fantasies activated by combat (Fairbairn, 1943; Leys, 1996). Although the term shell shock reflected a common understanding that the physical impact of blasts produced neurological effects independent of the "character" of the soldier, psychiatric observations soon undermined this thesis in ways that supported psychoanalytic thinking. Military doctors in field hospitals began reporting cases of war neurosis—for example, developing a paralyzed limb or becoming mute—after a relatively minor incident, such as falling into a ditch (Kinzie & Goetz, 1996). Further, doctors claimed that soldiers exposed to intense combat or held prisoner of war, even those buried alive, were less apt to develop the rigid nervous symptoms of the war neurotic. Whatever the approach, psychiatrists converged on the clinical significance of *volitional choice*—of the soldier feeling some degree of freedom to act—in the development of a war neurosis. More than the magnitude of a blast were the dynamics associated with the choice to fight or to flee.

In a historic psychoanalytic conference on the war neuroses in Budapest in 1918, the Hungarian psychoanalyst Sandor Ferenczi followed Freud's introductory remarks in addressing the delegates. Having served in the Austrian army as a doctor, Ferenczi, one of the intellectual heirs and intimates of Freud, expressed confidence that psychoanalysis was the victor in the battles over treatment of soldiers during the war years. He describes the vast scale of the war as a laboratory in the study of mental breakdown under conditions of emotional distress and fatigue. In *Remembering, Repeating and Working-Through*, Freud (1914/1958) locates the traumatic neurosis in the transfer of mental conflict into embodied action.

The patient does not remember anything of what he has forgotten and repressed, but acts it out. He reproduces it not as a memory but as an action; he repeats it, without, of course, knowing that he is repeating it.

(p. 150)

Ferenczi follows Freud's comments with a prognosis on the fate of post-war psychoanalysis:

> The mass-experiment of the war has produced various severe neuroses, including those in which there could be no question of mechanical influence, and the neurologists have likewise been forced to recognize that something was missing.
> (Ferenczi, Abraham, Simmel, & Jones, 1921, p. 6)

Although serving on the losing side of the war, Ferenczi claims victory for psychoanalysis in his remarks before the Congress. Shell shock had been jettisoned as a psychiatric term that failed to account for the psychic complexity of reactions to warfare. Among the burgeoning psychiatric terms produced by army doctors on the sides of both the Central Powers and the Allies, war neurosis was the one that carried the most currency. The delayed reactions of soldiers, emotional breakdowns that seemed unrelated to the immediate impact of war, seemed to support commanders' belief that soldiers routinely faked mental breakdown. Many became worse after evacuation from the front, which reinforced suspicions that soldiers were malingering. Shell shock was thought to be an acute emotional reaction and the "forward psychiatry" model of treatment—developed during World War I—was founded on a disciplinary model. Also described as the PIE model, forward psychiatry was based on proximity (P—treating soldiers close to their unit), immediacy (I—providing short-term care, typically warm food and rest), and expectancy (E—communicating authoritatively that the soldier must return to duty). When the pragmatic approach of forward psychiatry failed, physicians were summoned to produce more aggressive means of getting non-performing troops back on their feet (E. Jones & Wessely, 2014).

Ferenczi served in an army field hospital, assigned along with many other doctors the task of separating neuro-psychiatric cases from fakers and malingerers. Most suspect were those cases where there was a delayed onset of symptoms. The more immediate the reaction to an identifiable explosion or other event on the battlefield, the more credible the case of war neurosis. But many symptoms emerged weeks or months after exposure, giving rise to claims that the symptoms were fabricated. In describing such cases, Ferenczi compares the reactions of soldiers to those of a protective mother. "These injured men behave like the mother who rescues her child from danger which threatens its life with calm imperturbability and disregard of death, but faints after the act has been accomplished" (Ferenczi et al., 1921, p. 10). Just as the Great War opened cultural space for hysteria to migrate across the gender divide, the war destabilized gendered metaphors. Psychoanalysis emerged as one of those destabilizing sites.

## Doctors and Patients: *Folie à Deux*

The hysteric tells a story through her body, Freud and his colleague Joseph Breuer argued in a series of seminal papers during the 1890s (Breuer & Freud, 1893/1955). Rejecting the prevailing view that the hysteric suffered from an over-excited nervous system, Freud and Breuer explained how the hysteric used her body to communicate experiences that exceed ordinary language. Traumatic hysteria, through various formulations over the course of a century, has retained this idea of the body enlisted to communicate experiences that overwhelm the ego, and specifically the capacity of the ego to represent or symbolize highly disturbing events. During the war years, Freud continued to pursue a line of psychoanalytic thought that privileged the mind, and particularly forces of repression, over the impact of an external event in shaping the symptom picture (see Leys, 1996). But this emphasis on the body as a symbolic terrain for communicating mental conflict—as a canvas for the soul—remained a cornerstone concept that joined psychodynamic and medical approaches to the traumatic neuroses.

Freud overlooked, however, the role of the immediate audience in the performative language of hysteria. Physicians enlisted to pin down the pathophysiology of hysteria frequently commented on the elusiveness of the condition. The hysteric and her mutating symptoms entered the stage as a sort of Salome figure, staged early on as part of what physicians described as the seductiveness of the female hysteric. Charcot (1888) acknowledged his own struggles with the hysteric: "one finds himself sometimes admiring the amazing craft, sagacity, and perseverance which women, under the influence of this great neurosis, will put in play for the purposes of deception—especially when the physician is to be the victim" (p. 230).

During World War I, physicians were mobilized on both Allied and Central Powers sides and faced intense pressure to demonstrate allegiances to the war effort. Under mandates to produce quick cures, doctors may have unconsciously cued patients to exhibit increasingly dramatic symptoms. The symptoms told the story of soldiers who could not go on, but these symptoms did not protect soldiers from the charge of faking their conditions. Doctors routinely displayed patients and their symptoms to vivify their own powers to produce cures. The "feminine" position of the war neurotic—the basis of what Elaine Showalter (1985) describes as a crisis of masculinity generated by World War I—positioned psychiatric authority in relation to a helplessly ill subject. Treating soldiers carried this additional task of rehabilitating cultural ideals of manhood—of literally and figuratively getting men back on their feet.

Ferenczi and colleagues (1921) expressed an admixture of fascination, pity, and contempt that was characteristic of many doctors treating soldiers suffering emotional breakdowns. The medical fascination with female hysteria, and the implicit erotic voyeurism in the clinical gaze, failed to equip physicians with the emotional resources required in sorting out the troubles of distressed and defeated soldiers. "You all know those pathetic creatures who hobble along through the streets with shaking knees, uncertain gait and peculiar motor disturbances," Ferenczi offers to his audience, evoking the visual aspects of hysteria as spectacle:

> They give the impression of being helpless and incurable invalids; and yet experience shows that also this traumatic form of illness is purely psychogenic. A single treatment with electricity and suggestion, a few hypnotic settings are often sufficient in rendering these men capable of doing some work, if only temporarily and under certain conditions.
> (Ferenczi et al., 1921, p. 14)

Among the leading physicians of the Central Powers, Max Nonne, a neurologist from Hamburg, Germany, claimed center stage as a dominating figure. Hypnosis had gone into disfavor in the aftermath of scandals over Charcot's use of the method in treating hysteria at the Salpêtrière. The Great War ushered in a revival in the use of hypnosis in psychiatry, just as it would in World War II. The spectacle advanced beyond the still photographs lining the halls of Charcot's clinic, enlisting the new technology of movie cameras to provide verisimilitude to the cures on display. Nonne produced some of the more riveting moving pictures of shell-shocked soldiers of the war, and of his own commanding power over the display of their symptoms. In his silent film produced in 1916, after the turn to trench warfare, Nonne looms large over the bodies of palsied soldiers, with the figures of himself and the vulnerable patient set against a black screen that creates an eerie floating effect (Lewis, 2003; Schoefert, 2017). Some military commanders suspected that symptoms of war neurosis resulted from a contagion effect. Soldiers evacuated to military hospitals began to mimic one another in presenting the requisite symptoms to be relieved of duty. Since the scandal over Charcot in the 1880s, the contagion effect had suffered a disgraceful fate, usually discrediting both doctor and patient as performers.

The contagion effect reveals important psychological truths, however, about human social responses to suffering. The group culture of male hysteria during World War I, like Charcot's displays of female hysteria in the wake of the Franco–Prussian War, offers an important site for recognizing different ways of thinking about the body as a socially communicative register of distress. The discovery during Charcot's era of the performative aspects of hysteria, and how patients and doctors were cueing one another in the choreography of hysteria, invites a range of interpretations. One line of interpretation focuses narrowly on the symptom picture as a pathology located within the individual and analogous to a disease process. The question at this level often centers on whether the patient exhibits a real illness or a simulated one. Another approach widens the lens of interpretation to bring group influences or iatrogenic effects into the picture while also seeking to control such effects. Here the public health model of contagion effects and communicative diseases sensitizes observers to the transmission of mental pathology in groups.

But there is a third interpretive lens for framing these scenes. Identifications with a clinical profile can signify collective experiences of distress as well as forms of resistance and solidarity. Cultural codes regulate the use of the body in situations of extreme stress and trauma, just as they shape ritualized responses to grief and loss. Arlie Hochschild (1979) develops this same line of argument in describing the myriad ways humans conform to the demands of social situations in learning "feeling rules." Whether soldiers produced these dramatic symptoms to escape the horrors of battle, consciously or unconsciously, their embodied expression of distress was a necessary criterion for evacuation at the time. The pressures to return soldiers to duty intensified after the psychiatric casualties of Somme, one of the most horrific battles of World War I and the site of escalated trench warfare. This was where the most dramatic film footage of war neurosis was shot. While soldiers were undoubtedly stunned and overwhelmed by the terrors of that conflict, the specific language of that terror required, as it had during the American Civil War, a dramatic physical display of breakdown. As historian Peter Leese (2002) notes, doctors and patients mutually produced the symptomatology associated with the shell shock syndrome—and in ways that both accommodated and resisted military models of soldierly discipline.

## The Body and Its Lies

Alice Miller (2006), a leading author on psychic trauma, invokes one of the recurring rhetorical devices of the trauma therapy movement—the idea that trauma memory remains deeply buried in the psyche in ways that escape clinical detection. While trauma survivors may deceive themselves, "the body never lies."

Yet the body may indeed lie. Physical symptoms do not directly reveal underlying causes. The body registers emotional distress through physiological processes, but not in a way that translates into a straightforward nexus of causality. Medical specialists struggle with the ambiguities that arise in interpreting signs and symptoms no less than do psychological or psychiatric specialists. Van der Kolk (2015) cites neuroscientific findings to position PTSD as a valid disorder: "Since the early 1990s, brain-imaging tools have started to show us what actually happens inside the brains of traumatized people" (p. 21). Beginning with the hyper-aroused amygdala, van der Kolk traces the pathway of PTSD symptoms through regions of the brain, highlighting the hippocampus, thalamus, and cingulate. Whatever the brain structure or activity, the neuroscience findings cited by van der Kolk bolsters his basic story that the body—and the brain as one of the body's organs—signals the psychic truth of trauma.

Unlike the antipsychiatry movement of the 1960s and 1970s, the PTSD movement's revolt against psychiatry aimed more at entry into the medical diagnostic system than dismantling it. The struggle for the legitimacy of PTSD also meant expanding psychiatry to a widening populace of trauma survivors. Van der Kolk's medicalized portraits of PTSD echo the rhetorical strategies of earlier mind healers who divined hidden meanings in biological markers. Yet mind–body causal connections associated with PTSD symptoms remain an area of contested clinical speculations. In a 1994 review article on somatic complaints and PTSD, McFarlane and colleagues (1994) conclude with a call for greater attention to this nexus: "The degree to which certain physical symptoms are an integral part of the phenomenology of PTSD merits further research" (p. 724). A number of cross-cultural researchers argue that the body is enlisted in most cultures to express emotional distress (Kleinman, 1987; Porter, 1993). The World Health Organization cites gastrointestinal complaints as the most common psychosomatic disorder worldwide.

In a study of presenting complaints in primary care facilities in the United States, Javier Escobar (1995) and colleagues found that Central American immigrants had significantly higher rates of somatization than other ethnic groups. They also found that recent immigrants had lower rates of PTSD than US-born patients despite the immigrant patients' higher rates of exposure to war and trauma. The findings are based on structured PTSD interviews with patients seeking care at public hospitals. Estimating rates of PTSD in differing regional and cultural populations remain problematic, however, in that the questions themselves carry indeterminate political and cultural loadings. Take, for example, a set of items from the structured interview, asking patients to rate their responses on a scale from 0–4: "Have you experienced painful images or memories of combat or other trauma which you couldn't get out of your mind, even though you may have wanted to? Have these been recurrent?" This rating scale must seem strange as an artifact of American medical culture and its dissociative practices—its modes of simultaneously recognizing and disavowing suffering.

## Good Drugs/Bad Drugs

Psychiatrists are not reducible to virtuous or villainous, to either/or positions of healing or harming patients. Ethical guidelines for the clinical professions acknowledge that the two are intertwined—that the risk of harm inheres in many forms of treatment. For most contemporary psychiatrists, theories and speculations on mind–body relationships center on interactions associated with psychopharmacology. Yet, here too the clinicians' own struggles and sympathies enter the diagnostic picture. In the course of field research, I interviewed an Army major and psychiatrist who worked in a clinic in Kandahar, Afghanistan, and talked with him about his work. Hunched over the PC where he carried out his morning telemedicine consults, he explained the frustrations of doing psychiatry in a war zone. Since service members undergo drug screening during enlistment, many of them stop taking their meds. He said that he routinely asks soldiers having emotional reactions whether they were on psychiatric medications before coming into service. Although lying during enlistment is grounds for disciplinary action, the doctor was clearly sympathetic with these soldiers. Many had concealed their psychiatric histories and gone off their meds to get through the training. There is a long and noble history of men lying about their age or health problems to get into the military, he noted. Once in service, there is more latitude for prescribing drugs for mild anxiety and depression because these are conditions that can be attributed to combat or operational stressors. But some showed signs of more serious disorders. He had to weigh the risks of prescribing medications that could put service members and their units in danger against the risk of not treating the symptoms.

But the Army psychiatrist also framed psychoactive drugs as a disability rights issue. Many of these soldiers perform very well, he contended, and should be able to keep doing their jobs. The doctor complained about the limited pharmaceutical arsenal available to him in treating soldiers, which primarily involved helping them to get to sleep. He pointed out that drug use is inevitably part of warfare and that it's better to have controlled substances than the uncontrolled ones. Heroin, marijuana, and alcohol, key ingredients of the combat cocktail of the Vietnam era, are less available in these wars. Sniffing aerosol is one way that soldiers self-medicate, he adds, but it's a terribly toxic way of escaping the misery of a war zone.

Medical doctors have played leading roles throughout history in policing the boundaries between military-sanctioned and unauthorized use of mind-altering substances. During World War II, battle fatigue on both the Axis and Allied sides was managed through widespread distribution of amphetamines (Rasmussen, 2011). Since battle fatigue encompassed a loosely defined range of reactions, amphetamines served as drug of choice for a variety of ailments, including low morale. During the Civil War, morphine was synthesized and recognized as a vital aid in the treatment of battlefield trauma, even as morphine addiction emerged as a scourge following the war (Felbab-Brown, 2009).

Drugs that carry soldiers through casualties and dark nights on the battlefield generate moral panics as they circulate in the post-war home front (Kuzmarov, 2009). In the *Myth of the Addicted Army*, historian Jeremy Kuzmarov (2009) argues that drugs are a stand-in for more diffuse public anxieties over military missions. Repression of racial minorities has been carried out under the flag-waving crusades of the drug wars for decades, including in the military. Drug use acquired heightened signifying powers during the Vietnam War. Getting high could be a form of self-medicating, but it also connected troops with the cultural rebellions back home. As the military cracked down on marijuana use during the Vietnam War, destroying fields of marijuana cultivation, troops began to use heroin as a substitute because it was more readily accessible (Kuzmarov, 2009). In a study of drug use among returning Vietnam war veterans,

psychologist Lee Robins and colleagues (1974) report that although use of narcotics was a problem for some veterans, "heavy or addictive use was still much
rarer than might have been expected" (p. 39). The study was initiated after
government reports in 1971 that "drug use by United States service men had,
by all estimates, reached epidemic proportions" (Robins et al., 1974, p. 38).
As troops were being drawn down and thousands of men were returning each
month, government officials expressed alarm that veterans would contribute to
a wave of drug-related crime—and intensify what had already been declared as
a heroin epidemic among middle-class youth (Bentel & Smith, 1971). Robins
and colleagues (1974) note that the "narcotics virgin"—the service member
introduced to heroin in Vietnam—generated the gravest concern. The authors
conclude with a pointed criticism of forced treatment of veterans testing positive for narcotics. Thomas Szasz (1977) wrote a scathing commentary on the
mandatory drug treatment of soldiers returning from Vietnam as well, terming
the program a "pharmacological Gulf of Tonkin." He points out that drugs are
a ready-made scapegoat for failed public policies—and drug users in the military were the scapegoats for a war that was going badly.

Psychiatry occupies an ambivalent position in American culture as its
authorized drug dealers. Indeed, drug epidemics, including the opioid crisis
of the 2010s, often originate in the pharmaceutical industry and its aggressive marketing to physicians. Yet, psychiatry has undergone its own counter-
cultural movement since the 1990s as a visible cadre of physicians defends the
use of psychedelic drugs—a movement that has led to FDA and DEA trials
to establish the benefits of LSD and MDMA—Ecstasy—in the treatment of
PTSD. As psychoactive drugs promoted by pharmaceutical companies have
produced only modest results, with therapeutic benefits accompanied by worrisome side effects, psychiatrists in greater numbers have joined forces with proponents of psychedelics (Liechti, 2017; Sessa 2012b). Psychiatrist Ben Sessa
(2012a) claims that "the area where psychedelics show the greatest promise
is in enhancement of trauma-focused psychotherapy; in particular MDMA,
which can reduce the overwhelming fear response to memories of trauma and
improves engagement with therapy" (p. 201). And he offers his own diagnosis
of professional barriers: "After 100 years of modern psychiatry, our profession
is infected by learned helplessness. Unable to 'cure' our traumatised patients,
we treat them palliatively" (Sessa, 2018, para. 1). Much like conditioned dogs
that fail to venture out of their cages when offered a pain-free means of escape,
doctors are often fearful of venturing out of their own confining disciplinary
boundaries.

As I argue elsewhere in this book, trauma diagnoses carry a long history as
symptom-bearers of a deeper crisis of legitimacy in psychiatry. Public concerns
over addiction, over-prescribing, and chronic psychiatric conditions among
veterans in the 2010s open cultural space for treatments that would have been
unthinkable in the late 20th century with many of these treatments centering on
posttraumatic stress disorder. Unlike stimulants prescribed to keep warriors in

the fight, psychedelics are described as therapeutic in psychologically disarming veterans. In their capacity to reduce defensiveness, the drug fosters a visceral sense of connection with others, nature, and the universe. This advocacy and its pacifistic vision confront ideological barriers hardened through the long history of government campaigns demonizing psychedelics. But proponents have mounted informational campaigns to counter many of the over-blown claims issued by the government, including that psychedelic drugs cause war-related atrocities. PTSD advocates working with veterans in store-front clinics were among the most vocal critics during the Vietnam War era, among them psychiatrist Robert Jay Lifton. In *Home From the War*, Lifton (1985) disputes a Senate committee report that marijuana use was a leading cause of the My Lai massacre, adding that the real cause was the "atrocity-producing environment" of the war.

Founded in the mid-1980s, the Multidisciplinary Association for Psychedelic Studies, or MAPS, a non-profit organization, led a campaign to challenge legal restrictions to research on the therapeutic effects of psychedelics. Much like van der Kolk, founder Rick Doblin establishes the legitimacy of the drug for PTSD treatment on neuroscience. "It starts by reducing activity in the amygdala, which is the fear-processing part of the brain," he offers, going on to explain how the drug works "so that people's fearful emotions linked to trauma can be more easily recalled and processed" (Axelrod, 2018, para. 9).

The revival of psychiatric interest in psychedelics invites a closer look at the contributions of psychologist Timothy O'Leary as well, famous for advancing the mind-expanding benefits of LSD (see Greenfield, 2006). Based on psilocybin research carried out while he taught at Harvard in the early 1960s, Leary argued that the attitude of the experimenter toward the drug under investigation was a key factor in producing its observed effects. His "set-setting" hypothesis of drug effects included the attitudinal *set* of the researcher and the *setting* in which the drug is administered (Leary et al., 1965). When people have new sensory experiences, they look to external cues, including other people, for ways of interpreting those experiences. Many people had bad trips early on because they had not yet learned how to use hallucinogenic drugs nor had groups developed cultural practices around their use. The Harvard Psilocybin Research Project (PRP) looked to Indigenous knowledge and rituals around hallucinogens to build a critique of both American psychopharmacology and conservative ideas guiding much of the field of psychology. Leary, Litwin, and Metzger (1963) insist that "both everyday and scientific language are extremely inadequate for understanding altered states of consciousness" (p. 561).

The anti-psychiatry movement of the 1960s generated a critique of the medical model but it also embraced alternative states of mind. Interest in schizophrenia went beyond clinical control over disruptive symptoms to include learning from states of mind that radically departed from everyday perceptions. Non-psychotic people could learn from those whose minds were attuned to lower thresholds of disturbance in the society. In addition to the use of LSD for couples counseling in the 1960s, hallucinogens were used in a range of field settings. Leary and his colleagues (1965) describe a series of studies based on a treatment program in a correctional facility in Massachusetts. The study involved administering psilocybin to small groups of inmates who were invited to set their own goals for achieving insight. The set—the attitude of researchers—was explicitly positive in conveying an expectation of therapeutic growth. The setting—the immediate environment—offered a form of sanctuary within the prison: "During the session, the atmosphere is relaxed and permissive. Beds are provided for subjects to lie down if they wish, music is also available, the session is not interrupted by visitors or guards." More experienced prisoners from earlier phases of the study served as group leaders, "always ready to handle panic or paranoia by providing a warm, supportive 'reality' orientation" (para 17).

This study took place in the context of a larger anti-institutional movement—calls for more humane treatment of incarcerated persons. The reality orientation described by Leary invoked a critical sensibility resonant with many LSD enthusiasts today. In an interview with journalist Molly Oaklander (2018) on his research on psilocybin, Michael Pollen describes the settings conducive to its mind-altering effects:

> This isn't doctors giving you a pill and sending you out into the world. For a period of four or five hours, you are in a room that's decorated like a cozy den or study. You're lying down on a couch, you have eye shades on and headphones, which are playing a very carefully curated playlist to make you go inside to have an internal experience. And you're with two guides at all times, who are there looking out for your interests. It's an incredibly safe environment in which to let down your defenses, and that's essentially what happens.
>
> (para. 11)

Prior to the contemporary campaign to legalize LSD, one of the popular social signifiers of acid trips found its way into the DSM taxonomy and its list of PTSD symptoms. In the DSM-III-R (revised) published in 1987, flashbacks were listed as a symptom, even though there were scant references to flashbacks in the clinical literature on PTSD at the time. Brewin, Lanius, Novac, Schnyder, and Galea (2009) argue that what distinguishes PTSD from other anxiety disorders or depression are these "powerful multisensory image-based memories" thought to be "disconnected from contextual information" (p. 369). Intervening in disputes over the validity of PTSD as a clinical condition, the authors propose that PTSD diagnostic practices focus on this core phenomenon of "intrusive multisensory images accompanied by marked fear or horror" (p. 369).

Whereas hallucinatory states were embraced as doors to a wider world of perceptions by the anti-psychiatry movement, these same states enter trauma theory as merely registers of psychopathology. The idiom of the flashback in clinical culture drew on both LSD experimentation and film culture, and particularly on films featuring traumatized veterans (Luckhurst, 2008). In explaining the currency of the flashback idiom, Jerry Lembcke (1998) suggests that psychiatrists initially used the term loosely to describe anxieties veterans expressed in recalling their military service. Focusing specifically on the flashback, Roger Luckhurst (2008) claims that cinema helped "constitute the PTSD subject in 1980" (p. 177). The flashback combines the idea of suffering from reminiscences—the traumatic memory as an unbidden intrusion from the past—with the cinematic immediacy of altered perceptions. Unlike the palsied movements of the shell-shocked soldier, the flashback introduced a contemporary representational form for dramatizing the mental torments of veterans haunted by war memories. While the device had been used throughout the history of cinema, the flashback captured the public imagination through its enlistment of film culture and trauma theory to dramatize the intrusive power of war, brought under control through the combined powers of psychiatry and cinema.

As MAPS launches a new set of field trials on LSD and anticipates FDA approval for prescription use, it remains to be seen whether enthusiasm over psychedelics changes the minds of physicians. Most psychoactive prescription drugs end up on the streets, crossing the political border from good drugs to bad drugs. The therapeutic potential of psychedelics may depend on the kind of street culture that emerges as a counter to those VA hospitals on the hill.

## Conclusions

This chapter traces historical periods when the concept of psychic trauma achieved legitimacy through medical expertise. The dominant position of psychiatrists in the mental health field since the late 19th century rests on the medical training of doctors in reading physical signs, including indicators of trauma. The DSM-5 sought closer alignment with biological psychiatry in an effort to bring the mental health field more into alignment with medical knowledge and to overcome what DSM authors perceived as the vestiges of an old mind/body dualism. And there is some legitimacy to this claim. Unlike my own field of academic psychology, where disembodied cognitive theories prevail along with models of mind disconnected from sensuous human experience, psychiatry brings *soma* into the clinical picture. One of Freud's earliest and lasting contributions to psychiatry was in the idea that the symptom tells a story. He explained how repressed fears and fantasies could return through the disguised language of the body. Yet in *The Question of Lay Analysis*, Freud (1926) also cautions that medical training interferes with the listening skills required of psychoanalysts—that physicians are trained to bring the symptom under control rather than to be receptive to its manifold meanings for the patient.

Psychiatry achieved legitimacy as a profession through its expertise in translating ambiguous signs at the borders of existing medical knowledge. Many of these sites centered on the liminal concept of psychic trauma. Institutional recognition of psychic trauma often relied on an embodied performance of mental breakdown, often one that mimics a known medical disease, and on the healer's demonstrated power to restore functioning. As many of the cases of Charcot illustrate, medical theories of psychic trauma both widened and narrowed societal recognition of mental suffering. The First World War served as a key site for this widening of recognition. Psychiatrists achieved new prominence in diagnosing the conditions of soldiers suffering mental breakdowns. The concept of conversion hysteria, the prototypical war neurosis, protected some suspect soldiers from the heavy boot of military discipline. But this interpretation and its reliance on the transfer of conflict from the mind to the body offered little protection for the war resisters—for those who consciously refused to fight.

Even as psychiatric hospitals are less apt today to routinely use physical restraints, colonics or hydro-therapies than in the past, modern psychiatry provides chemical means of quieting those confined as rule-violators or as highly disruptive to others. The normalizing of prescribed psychoactive drugs for the mentally ill was accompanied in the 1960s by a pathologizing of recreational drugs, and particularly drugs used in poor communities. The medical marijuana campaign in the United States is instructive on this point. Through its demonstrated capacity to alleviate a number of chronic pain conditions, marijuana crosses a moral divide from deviant to therapeutic use—a divide heavily policed by the state and the medical profession. Marijuana dispensaries display an array of products, each with claims of unique benefits and catering to individual consumer tastes. The campaign shed its counter-cultural roots, including in Black and Latinx club scenes, to project a more sanitized image of healthy living, signified by the green medical cross and pharmaboutiques. While old white people can now legally smoke a bowl in many states to ease their aches and pains, blacks and other racial minorities continue to serve prison time for drug charges, including marijuana possession. As hallucinogens re-enter the psychiatric pharmacopeia, it remains to be seen how much their legitimacy will depend on professional experts and their clinical readings of altered states and expanded doors of perception.

The next chapter brings disability claims into my study of PTSD and traces the history of psychiatry as gatekeepers in the century-long medical task of separating "the truly ill" from "fakers and malingers." The PTSD movement subverted the old psychiatric typologies for sorting cases while at the same time introducing new categories that reproduced some of the same dilemmas.

# References

Alexander, F. (1932). *The medical value of psychoanalysis*. New York, NY: W. W. Norton & Co.

Alexander, F. (1950). *Psychosomatic medicine: Its principles and applications*. New York, NY: W. W. Norton & Company.

Ali, S., Jabeen, S., Pate, R. J., Shahid, M., Chinala, S., Nathani, M., & Shah, R. (2015). Conversion disorder—Mind versus body: A review. *Innovations in Clinical Neuroscience*, *12*(5–6), 27–33. Retrieved from www.ncbi.nlm.nih.gov/pmc/articles/PMC4479361/

American Psychiatric Association. (2013). *Diagnostic and statistical manual of mental disorders (DSM-5)*. Washington, DC: Author.

Axelrod, J. (2018, September 18). *MDMA, the main ingredient in ecstasy, could be key in helping veterans with PTSD* [News]. Retrieved February 23, 2019, from CBS News website: www.cbsnews.com/news/mdma-the-main-ingredient-in-ecstasy-could-be-key-in-helping-veterans-with-ptsd/

Bentel, D. J., & Smith, D. E. (1971). Drug abuse in combat: The crisis of drugs and addiction among American troops in Vietnam. *Journal of Psychedelic Drugs*, *4*(1), 23–30. https://doi.org/10.1080/02791072.1971.10471782

Breuer, J., & Freud, S. (1893/1955). On the psychical mechanism of hysterical phenomena: Preliminary communication from studies on hysteria. In J. Strachey (Ed.), *The standard edition of the complete psychological works of Sigmund Freud, volume II (1893–1895): Studies on hysteria*: Vol. *II* (pp. 1–17). London, UK: The Hogarth Press.

Charcot, J.-M. (1888). *Clinical lectures on certain diseases of the nervous system* (E. P. Hurt, Trans.). Philadelphia, PA: Davis.

Chester, A. C. (2007). The nose and sex: The nasogenital reflex revisited [Letter to the editor]. *Journal of the Royal Society of Medicine*, *100*(11), 489–490. https://doi.org/10.1258/jrsm.100.11.489-a

Connor, H. (2006). The use of anaesthesia to diagnose malingering in the 19th century. *Journal of the Royal Society of Medicine*, *99*(9), 444–447. Retrieved from www.researchgate.net/publication/321248538_The_use_of_anaesthesia_to_diagnose_malingering_in_the_19th_century

Crocq, M. A., & Crocq, L. (2000). From shell shock and war neurosis to posttraumatic stress disorder: A history of psychotraumatology. *Dialogues in Clinical Neuroscience*, *2*(1), 47–55.

Cryan, J. F., & Dinan, T. G. (2012). Mind-altering microorganisms: The impact of the gut microbiota on brain and behaviour. *Nature Reviews Neuroscience*, *13*(10), 701–712. https://doi.org/10.1038/nrn3346

Erichsen, J. E. (1867). *On railway and other injuries of the nervous system*. Philadelphia, PA: Henry C. Lea.

Escobar, J. I. (1995). Transcultural aspects of dissociative and somatoform disorders. *Psychiatric Clinics of North America*, *18*(3), 555–569.

Fairbairn, W. R. D. (1943). The war neuroses: Their nature and significance. *The British Medical Journal*, *1*(4284), 183–186. Retrieved from www.jstor.org/stable/20325356

Felbab-Brown, V. (2009). *Shooting up: Counterinsurgency and the war on drugs*. Washington, DC: Brookings Institution Press.

Ferenczi, S., Abraham, K., Simmel, E., & Jones, E. (1921). *Psycho-analysis and the war neuroses*. London, UK: The International Psycho-Analytical Press.

Freud, S. (1914/1958). Remembering, repeating and working-through. In J. Strachey, A. Freud, A. Strachey, & A. Tyson (Eds.), *The standard edition of the complete psychological works of Sigmund Freud, volume XII (1911–1913): Case history of Schreber, papers on technique, and other works: Vol. XII* (pp. 145–156). London, UK: The Hogarth Press.

Freud, S. (1921). Introduction. In E. Jones (Ed.), *Psycho-analysis and the war neuroses* (pp. 1–5). London, UK: The International Psycho-Analytical Press.

Freud, S. (1926). *The question of lay analysis: Conversations with an impartial person.* London, UK: WW Norton & Company.

Gilbert, S. M. (1983). Soldier's heart: Literary men, literary women, and the Great War. *Signs, 8*(3), 422–450. https://doi.org/10.2307/3173946

Goetz, C. G. (2011). The history of Parkinson's disease: Early clinical descriptions and neurological therapies. Cold Spring Harbor Perspectives in Medicine, 1(1), 1–15. https://doi.org/10.1101/cshperspect.a008862

Greenfield, R. (2006). *Timothy Leary: A biography.* Orlando, FL: Harcourt.

Guzman, I. P. (2018, November 28). How the body keeps the score: An interview with Dr. Bessel van der Kolk. *Brain World.* Retrieved from https://brainworldmagazine.com/how-the-body-keeps-the-score-an-interview-with-dr-bessel-van-der-kolk/

Haaken, J. (1998). *Pillar of salt: Gender, memory, and the perils of looking back.* New Brunswick, NJ: Rutgers University Press.

Hochschild, A. R. (1979). Emotion work, feeling rules, and social structure. *American Journal of Sociology, 85*(3), 551–575. Retrieved from www.jstor.org/stable/2778583

Jablensky, A. (1999). The concept of somatoform disorders: A comment on the mind-body problem in psychiatry. In Y. Ono, A. Janca, M. Asai, & N. Sartorius (Eds.), *Somatoform disorders* (pp. 3–10). Tokyo, Japan: Springer.

Jones, E., & Wessely, S. (2014). Battle for the mind: World War 1 and the birth of military psychiatry. *The Lancet, 384*(9955), 1708–1714. https://doi.org/10.1016/S0140-6736(14)61260-5

Killen, A. (2003). From shock to Schreck: Psychiatrists, telephone operators and traumatic neurosis in Germany, 1900–26. *Journal of Contemporary History, 38*(2), 201–220. https://doi.org/10.2307/3180655

Kinzie, J. D., & Goetz, R. R. (1996). A century of controversy surrounding posttraumatic stress-spectrum syndromes: The impact on DSM-III and DSM-IV. *Journal of Traumatic Stress, 9*(2), 159–179. https://doi.org/10.1002/jts.2490090202

Kleinman, A. (1987). Anthropology and psychiatry. The role of culture in cross-cultural research on illness. *The British Journal of Psychiatry, 151*(4), 447–454.

Kuzmarov, J. (2009). *The myth of the addicted army: Vietnam and the modern war on drugs.* Amherst, MA: University of Massachusetts Press.

Lacasse, J. R. (2014). After DSM-5: A critical mental health research agenda for the 21st century. *Research on Social Work Practice, 24*(1), 5–10. https://doi.org/10.1177/1049731513510048

Leary, T., Litwin, G., & Metzner, R. (1963). Reactions to psilocybin administered in a supportive environment. *The Journal of Nervous and Mental Disease, 137*, 561–573.

Leary, T., Metzner, R., Presnell, M., Weil, G. M., Schwitzgebel, R. K., & Winter, S. K. (1965). *A new behavior change program using psilocybin. Psychotherapy: Theory, Research & Practice, 2*(2), 61–72. https://doi.org/10.1037/h0088612

Leese, P. (2002). *Shell shock: Traumatic neurosis and the British soldiers of the First World War*. London, UK: Palgrave Macmillan.

Liechti, M. E. (2017). Modern clinical research on LSD. *Neuropsychopharmacology*, *42*(11), 2114–2127.

Lembcke, J. (1998). The "right stuff" gone wrong: Vietnam veterans and the social construction of post-traumatic stress disorder. *Critical Sociology*, *24*(1/2), 37–64. https://doi.org/10.1177/089692059802400104

Lerner, P. F. (1998). Hysterical cures: Hypnosis, gender and performance in World War I and Weimar Germany. *History Workshop Journal, 45*, 79–101.

Lewis, D. (2003). *Treatment of hysteria in WWI*. Retrieved February 23, 2019, from Dr Edmund Forester website: www.dredmundforster.info/treatment-of-hysteria-in-wwi

Leys, R. (1996). Death masks: Kardiner and Ferenczi on psychic trauma. *Representations*, (53), 44–73. https://doi.org/10.2307/2928670

Lifton, R. J. (1985). *Home from the war: Vietnam veterans: Neither victims nor executioners*. New York, NY: Basic Books.

Luckhurst, R. (2008). *The trauma question*. New York, NY: Routledge.

Mackenzie, J. (1920). A lecture on the soldier's heart and war neurosis: A study in symptomatology. *The British Medical Journal*, *1*(3093), 491–494.

Mayer, E. A., Knight, R., Mazmanian, S. K., Cryan, J. F., & Tillisch, K. (2014). Gut Microbes and the brain: Paradigm shift in neuroscience. *Journal of Neuroscience*, *34*(46), 15490–15496. https://doi.org/10.1523/JNEUROSCI.3299-14.2014

McCormick-Goodhart, M. A. (2012). Leaving no veteran behind: Policies and perspectives on combat trauma, veterans courts, and the rehabilitative approach to criminal behavior. *Penn State Law Review*, *117*(3), 895–926.

McFarlane, A. C. (2017). Post-traumatic stress disorder is a systemic illness, not a mental disorder: Is Cartesian dualism dead? *The Medical Journal of Australia*, *206*(6), 248–249. https://doi.org/10.5694/mja17.00048

McFarlane, A. C., Atchison, M., Rafalowicz, E., & Papay, P. (1994). Physical symptoms in post-traumatic stress disorder. *Journal of Psychosomatic Research*, *38*(7), 715–726. https://doi.org/10.1016/0022-3999(94)90024-8

Micale, M. S. (1985). The Salpêtrière in the age of Charcot: An institutional perspective on medical history in the late nineteenth century. *Journal of Contemporary History*, *20*(4), 703–731. https://doi.org/10.1177/002200948502000411

Miller, A. (2006). *The body never lies: The lingering effects of hurtful parenting* (Reprint edition and A. Jenkins, Trans.). New York, NY: W. W. Norton & Company.

Moscovich, M., Estupinan, D., Qureshi, M., & Okun, M. S. (2013). Shell shock: Psychogenic gait and other movement disorders—a film review. *Tremor and Other Hyperkinetic Movements*, *3*, 1–7.

National Research Council, & Institute of Medicine. (2007). *PTSD compensation and military service*. Washington, DC: National Academies Press.

Oaklander, M. (2018, May 16). This will change your mind about psychedelic drugs. *Time*. Retrieved from http://time.com/5278036/michael-pollan-psychedelic-drugs/

Porter, R. (1993). The body and the mind, the doctor and the patient: Negotiating hysteria. In S. L. Gilman, S. L. Gilman, H. King, R. Porter, G. S. Rousseau, & E. Showalter (Eds.), *Hysteria beyond Freud* (pp. 225–266). Berkley, CA: University of California Press.

Raese, J. (2015). The pernicious effect of mind/body dualism in psychiatry. *Journal of Psychiatry, 18*(1), 1–7. https://doi.org/10.4172/Psychiatry.1000219

Rasmussen, N. (2011). Medical science and the military: The Allies' use of amphetamine during World War II. *The Journal of Interdisciplinary History, 42*(2), 205–233.

Robins, L. N., Davis, D. H., & Nurco, D. N. (1974). How permanent was Vietnam drug addiction? [Supplement]. *American Journal of Public Health, 64*(12), 38–43. https://doi.org/10.2105/AJPH.64.12_Suppl.38

Roth, M. S. (1991). Dying of the past: Medical studies of nostalgia in nineteenth-century France. *History and Memory, 3*(1), 5–29. https://doi.org/10.2307/25618609

Schoefert, K. (2017, November 5). *Neurological narratives: War neuroses: Netley Hospital (1917)*. Retrieved May 3, 2019, from Neurovision website: https://neurovision.org.uk/videos/neurological-narratives-war-neuroses-netley-hospital-1917/

Sessa, B. (2012a). Shaping the renaissance of psychedelic research. *The Lancet, 380*(9838), 200–201. https://doi.org/10.1016/S0140-6736(12)60600-X

Sessa, B. (2012b). *The psychedelic renaissance: Reassessing the role of psychedelic drugs in 21st century psychiatry and society*. London, UK: Muswell Hill Press.

Sessa, Ben. (2018). The 21st century psychedelic renaissance: Heroic steps forward on the back of an elephant. *Psychopharmacology, 235*(2).

Shephard, B. (2003). *A war of nerves: Soldiers and psychiatrists in the twentieth century*. Cambridge, MA: Harvard University Press.

Shorter, E. (1997). *A history of psychiatry: From the era of the asylum to the age of Prozac*. New York, NY: John Wiley & Sons.

Showalter, E. (1985). *The female malady: Women, madness, and English culture, 1830–1980*. London, UK: Penguin Random House.

Stotland, N. L. (2008). Principles of psychosomatic medicine. In P. von Dadelszen & W. Stones (Eds.), *The global library of women's medicine*. Retrieved from www.glowm.com/section_view/heading/Principles of Psychosomatic Medicine/item/409

Szasz, T. S. (1977). Scapegoating "military addicts": The helping hand strikes again. In P. E. Rock (Ed.), *Drugs and politics* (1st ed., pp. 247–250). https://doi.org/10.4324/9780203792858-15

Terry, J. (2017). *Attachments to war: Biomedical logics and violence in twenty-first-century America*. Durham, NC: Duke University Press.

van der Kolk, B. (2015). *The body keeps the score: Brain, mind, and body in the healing of trauma* (Reprint edition). New York, NY: Penguin Books.

# Chapter 4

# Distressing and Disabling Conditions

Much like Franz Kafka, whose job as a claims adjuster by day shaped his outlook as a novelist by night, Veterans Affairs psychologists charged with disability cases suffer under the moral weight of their tasks. For Kafka, assessing claims for the Worker's Accident Insurance Institute in Prague led him to confront the problem of on-the-job injuries in factories, as well as to produce works centered on the arcane machinations of bureaucracies (Wagner, 2009). The bureaucrat administers rules with an even hand but can seem remote from the immediate anguish of plaintiffs. VA hospitals are often perched high on hills overlooking cities, and like Kafka's Castle, they serve as symbols of the administrative authority of the state in serving veterans of American wars.

My analysis of posttraumatic stress disorder began with questions concerning the progressiveness of this diagnostic category for mental suffering. This chapter looks at the diagnosis in relation to compensable grievances, an issue that enters into the economic currency of PTSD. A key thesis of this book argues that posttraumatic stress disorder operates defensively for professionals in a range of crisis situations and in response to conflicting institutional and political demands. The laws governing disability claims are an important part of that history. Beyond federal regulations governing disability claims, transference and countertransference reactions enter into the process—dynamics between assessor and claimant that are taken up in this chapter.

Disability claims represent a contentious area of the broader PTSD literature both because of the costs associated with compensation and the expansion in the late 20th and early 21st centuries of disability claims to include a wider range of conditions (McNally & Frueh, 2013). Benefits for veterans are based on disability rankings on a scale from 10 to 100 percent. The assessor typically assigns ratings in increments of 10 along that continuum. After hearing loss and tinnitus, PTSD is the most common basis for military-related disability claims (Crosby, 2017; Fagelson, 2007; McNally & Frueh, 2013), with most claims listing a number of additional diagnoses. While adding diagnoses may appear to be padding the file, this is not necessarily the case. PTSD is commonly associated with related mental health and medical conditions, many of which can be disabling.

The relationship between a mental disorder and functional impairments is inevitably multi-determined and depends on a range of contextual factors, including the level of social support (Ozner & Weiss, 2004). Indeed, the consequences of any given impairment, whether mental or physical, are contingent upon societal assumptions concerning normalcy. Disability rights activists have established "ableism" as a form of prejudice, re-mapping public spaces to expose oppressive structures that restrict the movements of disabled people, whether based on a mental health or intellectual or physical disability.

The PTSD movement of the 1970s and 1980s made significant gains in normalizing psychiatric symptoms as part of the predictable sequelae of warfare. Each era of military conflict has produced disabled veterans, many ushered onto ceremonial stages for political purposes. In many of these settings, the disabled veteran serves as sign of the injuries suffered by the nation. As a symbol of the valiant sacrifices born by the military, the impaired veteran has a longstanding place in the political imaginary. Sociologist Jerry Lembcke (1998) recounts the role of psychiatrists in creating a new kind of war hero: the emotionally disabled veteran fallen under the lethal weight of the US military machine. Citing a *New York Times* article during the 1970s, Lembcke outlines the psychiatric profile of the Vietnam War veteran suffering from PTSD: "They do not go berserk or totally withdraw. . . . Instead, they are bewildered, disillusioned, unable to cope" (p. 41). While the costs of warfare for the amputee or quadriplegic veteran are manifestly visible, those suffering mental symptoms confront a more daunting challenge in dramatizing the impacts of their military experience.

Since it was introduced into the DSM in 1980, the diagnosis of PTSD is increasingly cited in civil and criminal courts, employment cases, and veterans' compensation and benefits hearings. In this chapter, I show how this expansion in the use of the diagnosis has broadened psychiatry's role in the disciplinary regime of the modern state—a role that was critical to the rise of psychiatry in the 19th century as well. In the United States, controversy over disability claims has been most acute in political struggles over the long-term costs of warfare (Shulkin & Sheetz, 2019). McNally and Freuh (2013) explain how, "in an apparent effort to speed up the claims process, the federal government no longer requires documentation of exposure to a traumatic stressor for a veteran to qualify for PTSD" (p. 524). They describe a vicious cycle where the sheer numbers of veterans applying for disability based on PTSD makes questioning the grounds of these claims more difficult politically, leading to more pressure on the Veterans Disability Claims (VDC) system to streamline the process. One of the paradoxical effects taken up here centers on the silencing of many veterans in the process of granting their claims.

Psychiatric experts are central to these paradoxical effects in the courts as well as through the VDC. In tandem with the growth in veterans' disability claims are the armies of clinicians shaping their PTSD stories. The 1974 Federal Rules of Evidence changed the criterion for use of expert testimony, with relevance to fact-finding the key criterion rather than professional consensus on a particular diagnosis. Shuman (1995) argues that this new ruling promoted "expansive or creative interpretation of the diagnostic nomenclature" (p. 6). The storytelling skills of experts serve to bridge the massive and abstract scientific literature and the personal narrative, Shuman claims, with judges playing a gatekeeper role in determining competence and the relevance of expert testimony.

Mark Levy (1995) suggests that psychoanalysts are most often enlisted by defense attorneys as experts, less for their scientific credentials than for their storytelling skills and their training in converting symptoms into compelling personal accounts. This is not surprising given the emphasis in psychoanalytic theory on storytelling as a central feature of human development and consciousness (McDougall, 1974; Haaken, 1998, 2012; Haaken & O'Neill, 2014; Phillips, 2014). My interest here is in enlisting critical traditions of psychoanalysis to elucidate psychological and social dynamics involved in the production of PTSD diagnoses. Psychoanalysts can be as blind as other professionals to their tendencies to project a coherent narrative onto ambiguous signs and symptoms and to use clinical storytelling skills to advance self-interests. The stage for the work taken up in this chapter centers on assessment settings where experts are enlisted to establish causal links between a disturbing event in the past and a disabling condition.

## Battles on the Home Front

In the course of making the *Mind Zone* (Haaken, 2014) documentary, my crew and I filmed the 113th medical detachment as they were preparing to train and deploy at Joint Base Lewis–McChord (JBLM) in Washington state. Psychiatrists at Madigan Army Medical Center at JBLM, serving one of the most troubled military bases in the United States, came under heavy political fire in the early months of the following year. Anxieties had been mounting for some time over the alarming rates of suicide, domestic violence, and homicide on JBLM, where Madigan is housed (Yardley, 2012). The base extends over miles of land circled by towering northwest evergreens. Butter-yellow Scotch Broom shrubs, an invasive species that wipes out native vegetation, form a thick hedge around the base for much of the year. The massive Stryker vehicles, those eight-wheel tanks that transport thousands of infantrymen based at Lewis–McChord, are imposing in their projection of steely invulnerability. But parked under the towering trees, the tanks are dwarfed by this majestic setting, which survives the many soldiers that come and go, some never returning from their deployments or not returning as the same persons they were when they left. Behind the military structures and thickly forested terrain of the base, life at JBLM for enlisted soldiers and their families can be a living hell. The disturbing frequency of violence by soldiers at the base and several massacres by JBLM soldiers in Afghanistan put pressure on psychiatric teams to show they were getting the madness under control. The emotional toll of repeatedly deployed infantry captured the media in a storm of depressing reports (Brown, 2008; Scioli, Otis, & Keane, 2010)

But the controversy that unleashed a real firestorm of public outrage centered on a psychiatric forensic team at Madigan that denied hundreds of claims of soldiers filing for disability on the basis of service-related post-traumatic stress disorder (Murphy, 2012). The forensic team used the Minnesota Multiphasic Personality Inventory, a test that includes a scale for measuring faking symptoms, in their screening of claims. Among the 1,680 disability cases reviewed, some 690 had a PTSD diagnosis and 290 of those were subsequently denied (Bernton, 2012a). In defense of veterans whose claims were denied, some psychologists pointed out that the "F" scale (Faking) on this test did not generalize well to service members suffering from PTSD (Bernton, 2012a). Many may exaggerate their symptoms in order to feel recognized as suffering from a "real" condition, in part because military culture tends to maintain a high bar for expressing emotional distress (Bryan & Morrow, 2011). In addition to evidence of exaggeration and faking symptoms, claims were denied because the cases did not meet DSM criteria for PTSD. Debate among psychologists centered on whether soldiers differed from other groups on how many symptoms were required to meet the threshold criteria listed in the manual (Brewin, Lanius, Novac, Schnyder, & Galea, 2009). After the investigation, the Army released new guidelines that required more stringent evidence of false or exaggerated symptoms for purposes of financial gain.

Although questions about the generalizability of mental tests are everyday issues for psychologists, most of these discussions are carried out in dry academic journals or wonkish conferences. Forensic psychologists and psychiatrists—professionals trained to apply research findings to legal decisions—were blinkered by the day-to-day demands of their work without much awareness of the shortcomings of the tools they were using. They also were blindsided by the harsh spotlight of public accusations with their charges of gross failure to "care for our soldiers." The contested ground centered on the soldier's right to carry the label of PTSD as an honorable emblem of service. The media commentary charged that psychiatrists were implicitly ripping medals of honor from the uniforms of our infantry, and were grossly derelict in carrying out their duties (Bernton, 2012b).

A briefing for the evaluation team the prior year had included a list of lifetime payouts of up to $1.5 million per soldier disabled through the PTSD diagnosis (Bernton, 2012c). Some discussion had ensued over abuses of the psychiatric disability program, particularly with the liberalizing of criteria for making the diagnosis. Beyond establishing whether the traumatic event and symptoms met DSM criteria, the clinician also was required to evaluate "global functioning"—ratings of how much the person is impaired by the disorder in carrying out daily activities.

Ordinarily, conscientiousness over screening for abuses of the system would be the mark of a virtuous public servant. Indeed, case managers who administer workers' compensation, unemployment claims, or welfare benefits are routinely called out for lax oversight (MacGregor & Heilemann, 2017). Paranoid rage over welfare cheaters is the political bread-and-butter for many conservatives, pointing ecclesiastical fingers at those deemed fakers or lay-abouts. Yet Senator Patty Murray, a Democrat, arose in righteous indignation against the JBLM evaluators, leading the charge as the Chair of the Veterans Committee in demanding disciplinary action and review of the evaluators. The psychiatrists were placed on leave for the lengthy evaluation that ensued, after which they were reinstated. The review uncovered no evidence of denying claims based on budgetary concerns (Ruiz, 2013). Rather, denial of claims was based on the criteria established by the VA and Congress.

Instead, there was ample reason for concern over the sheer magnitude of disability claims being filed by veterans of the long wars. As of 2012, 45 percent of veterans of the wars in Afghanistan and Iraq had applied for service-connected disability compensation for psychiatric and nonpsychiatric medical problems and 28 percent had already secured benefits (McNally & Frueh, 2013). The sheer volume of disability claims generated puzzlement as well as alarm, particularly in that most were by service members without combat experience—the historical criterion for a PTSD claim.

The Veterans Affairs budget is separate from the Department of Defense, and VA staff often complain that the latter is far more apt to win Congressional support than the former. But the specter of hundreds of thousands of emotionally disabled veterans returning from the wars in Iraq and Afghanistan—and media reports of skyrocketing suicide rates—shifted the political focus from funding wars to funding their aftermath. In 2010, a Congressional Committee report, guided by their proclaimed duty to care for veterans, issued a bold reform in liberalizing criteria for PTSD disability claims. Previously only combat veterans—those directly engaged in fighting—escaped the lengthy bureaucratic process of filing for disability. But with the new rules, cases based on "operational stress"—conditions not directly related to combat—were also recognized. Further, there were changes in how traumatic stressors are documented. Under the new rules, the disability claim can be based on the veteran's account of the traumatic incident if supported by a VA psychologist or psychiatrist confirming that the incident did cause PTSD symptoms. This change added greater weight to the clinician's mental assessment. VA Acting Under Secretary Walcoff explains that the regulation will eliminate the need to search for records to verify veterans' accounts, "often a very involved and protracted process," and will enable VA officials "to move more quickly to award more benefits to veterans suffering from PTSD" (Wilson, 2010).

The legislation was part of a trend underway in expanding disability benefits. The Wounded Warrior Assistance Act and the Dignified Treatment of Wounded Warriors Act, both passed unanimously in the Senate in 2007, raised the ceilings on disability payments. By the tenth year of the long war, over 400,000 service members were receiving disability payments, with PTSD a leading basis for claims (McNally & Frueh, 2013).

Advocates for women in the military had for years challenged the combat criterion, arguing that tying so many benefits to combat experience produced a bias against female service members (Murdoch et al., 2003). The military sexual trauma (MST) campaign, taken up again later in this chapter, drew attention to the minefield of threats female service members navigated. But it also gathered momentum through complaints over the combat bias in access to disability benefits—a complaint that resonated as well with many male service members and the majority of the armed services without direct combat experience.

The changing landscape of warfare, with the shifting military missions associated with the Iraq and Afghanistan wars, also contributed to change in the combat criterion. Service members without infantry training routinely traveled in convoys that could be subject to attack from an improvised explosive device (IED). Risks of lethal violence were not distributed along the same axis of a "front" and "rear" as they had been in World War II, when the disability laws were established. Furthermore, female service members were engaged in risky operations not formally recognized by the military as involving combat.

Yet there was uneasiness that some veterans were gaming the system and that the disability program was producing chronic PTSD as a socially cultivated malady (Gade, 2013; Harbaugh, 2017). Much like other benefits programs, bureaucratic mechanisms are in place for sorting legitimate from false claims. But, unlike workers compensation or accident cases, where courts set high bars for awarding damages to plaintiffs, the problem of illegitimate veterans' claims confronts anxieties on many fronts. And the threat of failing to "support our troops" hangs particularly heavy over the heads of examiners.

Critics of the VA disability system argue that an earlier era of denial concerning post-war mental conditions has been overtaken by a reactive and pathogenic system of indulgences. In noting the 300 percent increase in disability claims of veterans of the Iraq and Afghanistan conflicts, Frueh and colleagues (2007) offer their sobering assessment: "We may be instilling counterproductive social expectations that war-zone deployment will make veterans psychiatrically disabled, potentially a self-fulfilling prophecy" (p. 2144). The authors base their argument on data suggesting that veterans seeking mental health services through the VA have a disincentive to benefit from treatment and that the low rates of recovery from PTSD among veterans is an artifact of the disability system.

## The Claims Assessor

Psychologists and psychiatrists serve as both evaluating and treating clinicians, although these are different positions within the VA system. Clinical services at the VA are separated from the process of evaluating disability claims because professional ethics guard against such dual roles, particularly where there are conflicting interests. But in the minds of veterans, these two arms of the VA system are tightly folded together because the review process depends on evaluation of the claim, including military record, and the current diagnosis and treatment. And while the evaluator and treatment positions are organizationally separate, the VA culture contributes to the blurring of boundaries. If patients improve and clinicians chart their therapeutic progress, the veteran is more likely to lose his/her disability claim. Once awarded, however, disability awards are not affected by participation in treatment. Indeed, participation in PTSD treatment tends to decline after the awarding of disability claims (McNally & Frueh, 2013).

Worthen and Moering (2011) note the lack of adequate VA staff for properly conducting mental health disability evaluations. In 2011, the VA began permitting private providers, primarily psychologists and psychiatrists, to conduct exams with the VA's new Disability Benefits Questionnaire (DBQ) system. The authors offer an accompanying caveat, however: "The DBQ form is deceptively simple. Beware of the temptation to tell a veteran that you can interview him or her in a standard 50-min session and then check off the DBQ boxes" (p. 192). The authors describe pressures on VA clinicians to speed up the process since PTSD applications became eligible for fast-tracking in the system (Wadsworth, n.d.). Clinicians are often allowed only an hour for an exam even though the professional norm for forensic evaluations is from three to eight hours. The case file includes a statement written by the veteran—their story of what happened and how it affects their current functioning—as well as testimony by family members, friends, and military comrades.

Acknowledging emotional distress for assessors, Worthen and Moering (2011) add sympathetically that the letters can be "heart-wrenching" (p. 195). They note the difficulties in bringing test scores into alignment with VA policies as well. Instruments designed to detect faking or feigning are problematic because they do not "give the veteran the benefit of the doubt" in areas of irreducible ambiguity—a policy requirement of the VA disability evaluation system (p. 197). Nonetheless, Worthen and Moering insist, VA psychologists carry a professional duty to assess for malingering. The authors observe that "there is so much resistance to screening for dissimulation within the VA that we feel compelled to make a strong, detailed case for its importance" (p. 202). While some clinicians mistakenly view the compensation as "an *entitlement* program, i.e., one that awards benefits for a veteran's service in a combat zone," the system is in actuality "an *indemnity* program in which the VA provides benefits to veterans who have suffered occupational impairment as a result of their psychology [sic] injury" (p. 188).

Yet many veterans *do* see disability benefits as an entitlement program. The website Hadit.com—founded in 1997 and one of the most commonly used non-VA sites for pension and compensation questions—makes this distinction explicit. Parodying the Soldier's Creed, which begins with "Leave no comrade behind," the tagline reads: "Leave No One Behind—Not on A Jungle Trail; Not on A Desert Trail; Not on A Paper Trail." Under testimonials, veterans express their outrage and valiant struggles with the VA, and their solidarity with others on the site:

> Hadit.com has information that the VA doesn't want you to have. The information on hadit.com led me to a 90% rating and a clear path to 100%. With hadit.com you do not need a VSO to file your claim. Trust hadit.com and get the rating you truly deserve and not the rating the VA gives you to balance their budget.
>
> The VA benefits are yours, you EARNED them. They are not a handout or charity. It is OUR Veterans Affairs. It belongs to you, not the government or the VA. Contrary to what the VA tries to do to the Veteran and the roadblocks and minefields they use to try to discourage or stall the Veteran, it is OUR VA.

The distinction between the government and a beloved entitlement program ("OUR Veterans Affairs") often arises in conservative political rhetoric (e.g., "Keep government hands off my Medicare!"). The Department of Veterans Affairs is, of course, a government program, established in the 1920s to provide pensions and medical, psychiatric, and rehabilitative care for World War I veterans. But the VA as an institution is very much a product of veterans' struggles as well, including in its early formation. During the economic crisis of the 1920s, veterans marched on Washington, camping out for months to protest the government's failure to pay bonuses promised after the war. When protestors rioted at the Capital, President Hoover sent in troops to restore order. Although the protestors did not win the bonus payments, the uprising eventually contributed to political momentum for the passage of the GI Bill—a benefits package that supported the transition of 16 million World War II veterans (Dickson & Allen, 2006).

For many veterans, the disability program may indeed be a kind of "war bonus"—the signifier of sacrifice and safety net in a highly competitive economy (Zarembo, 2014). After a deployment, veterans find that the job they return to may not be the same one that they left, or that their military occupational specialty (MOS) does not translate into opportunities on the home front (Shay, 2003).

## Doctors, Disability, and Railway Spine

Forensic psychologists are more apt to focus on industrial accidents than warfare in tracing their own intellectual history. The prototypical forensic case for PTSD centers on one of the primary engines of industrial expansion in the 19th century—the railroad—and a condition called *railway spine*. In the last chapter, the condition was taken up as a site for competing claims and medical expertise centered on psychic trauma. But the condition holds an important place in the history of disability claims and workmen's compensation laws as well (Loughran, 2009). Wolfgang Schivelbusch (1979) describes how the rash of railway spine cases in Europe in the late 19th century arose after the Continent had psychically and culturally integrated the railroad into modernity. The claim seems counter-intuitive in that these cases were *less* common during the early phase of the railroads than during the later period when they were established as a mode of transportation. On a collective level, Schivelbusch suggests, the condition may be interpreted as a "return of the repressed"—a reaction to a world that had been profoundly transfigured over the course of decades. The railroad in the 19th century occupied a vivid and emotionally charged site in the social imaginary—a site of threat and danger, but also of mobility. Whereas the soldier emerged as the symbolic bearer of violent colonial conquests in the 20th century, the traveler occupied this liminal position in the prior century. And, indeed, rail accidents were quite common. As Schivelbusch points out, news of a railway accident served as an uncanny awakening of the violent force of the locomotive and the impotence of human efforts to manage its powers.

The rise of medicine and the authority of physicians, and particularly those at the border between neurology and psychiatry, came onto the political stage through their role as adjudicators of railway spine, typically manifested by debilitating weakness and anxiety after either witnessing or being victim of a train accident. A puzzling feature of the condition was the absence of physical signs of injury. By the 1860s, railway companies were paying damages to victims without a medically established cause, but the medical rationale required a new theory of trauma—one that mapped onto prevailing medical thinking. In one of the early studies of railway spine, published in 1867, John Eric Erichsen describes the heated atmosphere of the debates:

> There is no class of cases in which medical men are now so frequently called into the witness-box to give evidence in courts of law, as in the many intricate questions that often arise in actions for damages against railway companies for injuries alleged to have been sustained by passengers in collisions on their lines, and there is no class of cases in which more discrepancy of surgical opinion is elicited than in those now under consideration.
>
> (p. 18)

Claims based on industrial accidents have tended to involve physical disabilities more commonly than emotional trauma. The cases of railway spine are striking because victims exhibited a feature commonly associated with war neurosis. One of the key features was the delay in symptoms until long after exposure to the accident. Delayed reactions to stressful events have long been observed in the scientific literature. But doctors were summoned to provide a medical explanation for the physiological pathway of such effects. Debates ensued among physicians over whether the "softening of the spine"—the body part that emerged as site of etiological explanation—led to a gradual weakness that overtook the victim. The causes of railway spine were strenuously debated. One area of agreement among physicians—whether taking the position that the condition was somatic or psychological—was that even relatively minor shocks could produce dramatic delayed effects.

The late 19th-century neurologist Jean-Martin Charcot, whose work was taken up in Chapter 3, is credited with bringing psychic trauma onto the medical stage as a basis for the condition of hysteria. He demonstrated that the symptoms of hysteria induced by trauma conformed to a predictable medical pattern of illness. Lesser known is Charcot's early career as a claims evaluator for a French railway company. In securing legitimacy for hysteria as a psychogenic illness, Charcot (1888) drew on his prior career as an evaluator of railway spine cases:

> Quite recently, male hysteria has been studied in America by Putnam and Walton, principally in connection with and as a sequel of traumatisms, and more especially of railroad accidents. They have recognized along with Page, who has also interested himself in this question in England, that many of those nervous accidents designated under the name of *railway spine*, which, in his opinion, might better be called *railway brain*, are in reality, whether appearing in man or in woman, simply hysterical manifestations.
>
> (p. 99)

Charcot uncoupled hysteria from gender, while also attempting to uncouple hysteria from suspicions of fakery. Charcot argued through clinical cases that men were as vulnerable to hysteria as women, even though it was not until World War I that the specter of men breaking down in staggeringly large numbers took center stage. The development of neurology as a specialty, and later psychiatry as a separate field from neurology, flourished in this forensic climate where claims and counter-claims over the maladies of modern life and interpretations concerning hidden motives and mysterious illnesses were being adjudicated.

## Psychiatry, Disability, and the Law

As a forensic diagnosis, PTSD occupies a tense border between medicine and the law. As Mark Levy (1995) notes in looking back on the early years following inclusion of PTSD in the DSM manual, the diagnosis "flourishes today in a medical–legal climate where Post-Traumatic Stress Disorder (PTSD) claims comprise a substantial and costly portion of personal injury and employment litigation" (para. 1). Researchers also raise alarms over the "rising tide" of workers enlisting the diagnosis in compensation cases. Stone (1993), for example, claims that bringing PTSD into the DSM system became a "lightning rod for a wide array of claims and disturbances" (p. 17). No other diagnosis has had such an impact on the legal system, he declares. And for experts summoned on behalf of insurance companies, there is an array of dismissive labels for claimants pursing psychological damages, from "thin skulls" to "egg shell psyches" (Calandrillo, 2006; McQuade, 2001). In legal parlance, these terms are deployed to argue that vulnerabilities or weaknesses in the claimant are the real cause of the alleged breakdown in functioning. Some courts have agreed to review "thin skull" cases on the grounds that preexisting conditions need not nullify the damaging effects of a traumatic accident. But in general, preconditions work against plaintiffs, even though PTSD represents the ideal plaintiff prototype because it argues that a single event can cause dramatic disruptions in functioning even after a delayed period of time.

Koch, Douglas, Nicholls, and O'Neill (2006) offer a broader historical explanation for the increase in compensation claims after the introduction of PTSD into the DSM in 1980. Historically, civil courts had been reluctant to award damages for emotional injury. A rigid dualism governed the courts in separating mind and body until the PTSD era. The thinking was that people are generally psychologically thick-skinned. Psychological harms continue to be argued through the legal discourse of injury, however. This explains in part the use of brain and physiological markers of PTSD in claiming its legitimacy (van der Kolk, 2002), as well as the more recent language of "moral injury" in describing psychological impacts of war (see Nash & Litz, 2013; Shay, 2014). While jurisdictions in the United States varied considerably in their rulings, there was a general liberalizing trend in the 1980s in awarding emotional damages, particularly if the temporal proximity of accident and symptoms could be established.

The forensic history of PTSD is both cause and effect of these broader social struggles, including alliances between mental health practitioners and defense attorneys. The literature on the moral injuries of war, intended to widen PTSD beyond the medical model, draws heavily on the legal prototype for emotional harm. Injuries denote externally imposed destructive impacts. Demonstrating such impacts generally relies on observable indicators.

Trauma therapists also rely heavily on the proximal cause rule that governs legal adjudication of PTSD cases. It becomes more difficult to establish proximal causality, however, as time expands between the traumatic event and subsequent symptoms. The recovered memory phenomenon of the 1990s, taken up again in the next chapter, was in part a response to this requirement of temporal proximity and statutes of limitations on making claims. The anti-war and anti-sexual assault movements were able to establish causal connections between a traumatic event in the past and later onset of symptoms by arguing that the legal clock starts when the victim becomes conscious of the traumatic memory. The mechanism of dissociation was enlisted to bridge this temporal gap and to explain how traumatic memory could be stored relatively intact in mind but out of consciousness until a later event revived the memory. As Mark Levy (1995) argues:

> The recent sea change in our cultural and social attitudes has resulted in an epidemic of psychological injury claims not only in connection with personal injury suits but also as a by-product of "repressed memory/false memory" hysteria. . . . Among the various psychiatric diagnoses found in psychological injury claims, the major stress diagnosis, PTSD, is one of the most highly compensated.
>
> (para. 2)

PTSD and delayed memory were effective strategies in the legal advancement of victim claims. Victims in situations where they are dependent on their abusers are often unable to conceptualize what has happened to them, much less act on what has happened, until they have achieved a level of emotional safety and maturity. Based on this line of argument, advocates were able to effectively challenge statutes of limitation, particularly in cases of childhood sexual abuse.

The delayed memory phenomenon was important on this legal front even though research on memory increasingly demonstrated the malleability of recollections. In the early PTSD movement, however, the concept of delayed memory of military trauma operated as a discursive strategy in countering collective denial over the long-term effects of warfare. Veterans and sexual abuse survivors were, in a sense, symptom bearers for a society suffering from its own form of cultural amnesia concerning the pervasive violence produced by the state. As these same rhetorical strategies were tested in the courts or assessment settings, the factual grounds of the cases took center stage. The signifying power of delayed memory as a rhetorical device—the role of psychiatric symptoms as bearers of the repressed stories of the culture—suffered numerous defeats under the obsessive rules of the judicial system.

In previous chapters, I have shown how PTSD is most commonly used in contexts where conflict arises over social distribution of responsibility for emotional suffering. The diagnosis is more apt to be assigned in settings involving the courts, such as state psychiatric hospitals or criminal and civil cases, as well as in veterans' facilities. Mental health professionals take on this role of assessing states of mind involved in adjudicating cases. Since wars are the laboratories of history where stress conditions have been most consistently documented, the battlefield has acquired a unique status as incubator of traumatic stress. In searching for the precursors of PTSD, military historians tend to cite psychiatric conditions that flourished during previous wars, from nostalgia, soldier's heart, battle fatigue, and shell shock to war neurosis.

Forensic psychologists and psychiatrists, however, present a different genealogy of PTSD—one that reveals a darker side to professional framing of psychic trauma. In the introduction to *Post-Traumatic Stress Disorder in*

*Litigation*, Ralph Slovenko (2003) traces the history of emotional trauma claims through pejorative terms leveled against plaintiffs, from compensation neurosis, industrial neurosis, accident neurosis, and pension neurosis to secondary gain neurosis. Unlike the war neurosis, which carried notes of sympathy for emotionally vulnerable soldiers, forensic diagnoses in accident cases were meant to disqualify plaintiffs, often casting them as frauds. Bonnie Green and Stacy Kaltman (2003) offer definitions of the key terms: "The terms accident neurosis and compensation neurosis have been used to suggest that a condition (e.g., PTSD) for which compensation is sought will resolve once the litigation is settled" (p. 32). Suspicion of faking symptoms is generally part of litigating emotional damages, although courts in recent decades have widened legal ground for emotional suffering and pain, particularly if emotional damages are attached to bodily harm, for example, paralysis (Gold, 2003).

Slovenko (2003) explains the affinity between the diagnosis of posttraumatic stress disorder and forensic reasoning: "PTSD is a favored diagnosis of plaintiffs because the DSM sets it out as incident specific. It tends to rule out other factors important to the determination of causation," such as a diagnosis of depression, which "opens the issue of causation to many factors other than the stated cause of action" (p. xxiv). He adds that the PTSD diagnosis tends to evoke sympathies from juries and judges because the sufferer is not implicated in the development of the condition.

## Post-War Grievances

An oft forgotten history of psychiatric involvement in war-related trauma involves adjudicating *post-war* claims. In her analysis of medical records related to veterans following World War I in France, Patricia Prestwich (2003) identifies a pattern of consistent reluctance among doctors to authorize veterans' mental disability claims, in spite of public sympathy for disabled veterans. Medical investigations for reports to the Pension Boards included questioning family and neighbors about pre-war adjustment and probing for family histories of insanity that would invalidate war-related claims. Prestwich notes the widespread public support for the disability reports of veterans: "The responses from families and communities were both coherent in their definition of mental illness and categorical in their belief that the only possible explanation for the disturbed behavior of veterans was the horror of war" (p. 249).

Wars produce vast bureaucracies in carrying out short- and long-term missions and spawn an array of psychological training programs, many through the VA system. Public solidarity with veterans after wars leads to legislation favoring benefits programs, from housing and educational benefits to advantages in employment opportunities. The specter of disabled veterans also generates anxiety and guilt, some of which lends support to public programs to keep veterans out of sight. The Veterans Administration Health Care system in the 1920s grew in part from public uneasiness in witnessing so many home-less veterans on the streets of America (J. Sardo, personal communication, May 16, 2011).

Historian Jennifer Mittelstadt (2015) describes the decades-old dilemma for the military in countering associations between the army—the largest of the five branches—and social welfare. The transition in 1973 to an all-volunteer military was achieved through generous benefits and supports from housing and pensions to extensions of the GI Bill for schooling. Mittelstadt notes that "it was no coincidence that the army's hesitation concerning its support system emerged in the late 20th century at the same time that President Bill Clinton promised to 'end welfare as we know it'" (p. 173). Many veterans' services began to be outsourced and privatized, from health care and counseling to housing and employment services.

One risk of war—untallied in war planning—involves the potential for rebellions among the troops on return. The Civil Rights Movement grew in part out of the experiences of soldiers fighting for freedom abroad and then facing the expectation to relinquish those same freedoms at home. Government campaigns to mobilize women workers during World War I and II valorized untapped female strengths and stressed the necessity of departures from nor-mal gender roles required by the war effort. As Margaret Higonnet and Patrice Higonnet (Higonnet, 1987; Higonnet & Higonnet, 1987) argue in their history of post-World War gender relations, many women resisted the restoration of the old patriarchal order after men returned home, but they lacked the political power to fight back. Military experience for men, as well, generates desires and possibilities taken into the post-war world—states of mind that may also produce bitter disappointments.

A striking feature of American discourse on veterans' benefits is the special status the armed services member acquires as one who can reasonably make claims on the state. As most politicians can attest, public campaigns to cut veterans benefits are off limits. With the transition to an all-volunteer military after the Vietnam War, mental health teams were increasingly integrated into Defense Department planning to keep service members feeling good enough about the military to re-enlist (J. Sardo, personal communication, June 2, 2011). And as a smaller percentage of the American public serves, public identifications with the military become less based on shared responsibilities and notions of citizenship. The liberalizing of PTSD criteria grants veterans a license to claim hardships, a form of pay-out for service, without the burdens of listening to their complaints. The experts whose job it was to listen long enough to act on Congress's approval of millions in increased disability pay-ments were assigned this ethos: "At the Department of Veterans Affairs, we take care of heroes, because they fought for us" (D. Green, 2016).

Beyond disability benefits and VA medical and psychiatric services, a range of special veterans' programs sprang up during the wars in Iraq and Afghanistan, from Hire a Hero incentive programs for employers, the Give an Hour network of therapists offering counseling services, special courts for criminal and civil cases involving veterans, and programs focused on housing and homelessness. While many of these same services are available for veterans elsewhere in the world, social services tend to be integrated into the larger social welfare systems in other advanced industrial countries (Crabb & Segal, 2018). In their analysis of international data, military sociologists Crabb and Segal (2018) conclude that "the United States is generally understood to provide less social welfare through government transfer programs than governments in Europe" (p. 74). They go on to explain that veterans' benefits, particularly since World War II, represent the largest exception to this pattern and that "large-scale veterans benefits are uniquely American" (p. 74). Yet political discourse on veterans' programs routinely distinguishes them from welfare, with its politically stigmatized associations with dependency on the state. The disavowal of dependency needs within military communities, even as the armed services do appeal to dependency needs in its recruitment programs, leads to a return of the repressed in outraged veterans.

In PTSD assessments, however, struggles over dependency needs are notably absent on check-lists of symptoms. Ronald Fairbairn (1943), discussed in the last chapter, described psychoneurotic conditions among troops as a symptom of infantile dependencies. From his perspective, soldiers broke down on the battlefield because they refused to grow up. This pathologizing of vulnerability and dependency—and the correlative idealizing of illusions of masculine autonomy—may be the real story behind the disabling side of the PTSD diagnosis.

The 2012 debate in Congress over disability rights—and refusal to ratify the United Nations Convention on the Rights of Persons with Disabilities (Blanchfield & Brown, 2015; Montopoli, 2012)—serves as one of many indicators of the vast distance between claims of veterans and those of other groups with special needs. One of the benefits of disability awards involves access to VA services. For Reserve or Guard members, access to VA services ends after a brief post-deployment period. With a for-profit health care system in the United States, the Veterans Administration serves as the only version of socialized medicine in the country and is one of the largest socialized health care systems in the world. Although a source of bitter outrage for many veterans, the VA system is highly praised as well. A comprehensive study by the Rand Corporation concluded that the VA performed at higher levels than the private health care system on almost all measures (Asch et al., 2004).

## Detecting Deception

In a King's College conference in London on oral history from World War II, Simon Wessely (2005) set the thematic tone for the conference by suggesting that "war stories change according to who is doing the telling, who is doing the listening, and why the story is being told" (p. 473). Professionals assessing

PTSD claims are trained to enlist scientific procedures to control for their own subjective responses, as well as to ferret out the subjective distortions of claimants. Although screening for malingering is standard practice in civil and criminal cases involving PTSD, the introduction of the diagnosis into the DSM in 1980 ushered in proscriptive inhibitions concerning open discussion of deception. Trauma therapists routinely called for "believing the victim" as part of treatment, which translated into taking the presenting story at face value. Trauma therapists caution against re-traumatizing the patient by questioning the account, with believing the victim listed as the first principle of clinical care. At the same time, the DSM manual warns that the diagnosis may be easily simulated and deployed for financial gain (American Psychiatric Association, 2013). For the evaluator, documenting the trauma history and matching the index event to the symptom picture can be daunting indeed.

Clinicians carry the task of untangling the threads of these stories and of separating the way everyday people elaborate on personally meaningful memories from outright faking. Kenneth Morel (2010), a psychiatrist working in the VA system, has amassed an array of psychometric tools for identifying fakers, along with standard guidelines for the clinical interview. In issuing guidelines, he cautions against endorsing too readily the PTSD story based on sympathy for the veteran's expressed need. Morel offers examples of colleagues stating, "I gave the patient a diagnosis of PTSD because he really needs the money" (p. 34). Financial need is one of the main criteria for accessing VA health and mental health services—and access to VA services is the standard payout for a 10 percent disability rating. One way of describing the disability system is that it expands the reach of the VA health care system to those otherwise not covered. Indeed, most veterans with stable employment and health care benefits do not use the VA system. One expression of the social class dynamics of veterans' services emerges in oblique references to "trouble paying the bills."

Morel (2010) hones in on specific pitfalls in focusing on the vet's trauma story and symptoms rather than on the question of how those symptoms affect current functioning. "Perhaps the most overlooked criterion for a diagnosis of PTSD is criterion F," he suggests, the criterion for the diagnosis that requires establishing "significant impairment in social and occupational functioning of the patient" (p. 23). While Morel cites evidence of the tendency among veterans to exaggerate their symptoms, he adds that the more critical issue centers on how symptoms affect capacities to carry out roles and tasks in daily life, from family and interpersonal domains to finding and keeping employment. A disability rating does not mean that the person cannot function in these roles. A score of 50 percent disability, for example, allows that the person may be employable but requires support services or accommodations.

In recognizing the many gray areas that arise in clinical assessment for PTSD, Morel (2010) presents an array of psychometric tools available for evaluators. Much of the problem, he suggests, lies in clinicians' reluctance to probe for further detail or order military records to verify service-related incidents, or to follow-up with psychological testing. The military code requires solidarity with service members—"leaving no comrade behind." VA clinicians—many serving as reservists in the military—often express uneasiness that disability judgments do indeed leave many veterans behind. However, the disability system does grant veterans the benefit of doubt in ambiguous situations, requiring that the claimed traumatic stressor is "more likely than not" to have caused the presenting symptoms.

VA clinicians feel the pressure of honoring vets, even as they recognize their own collusion in protecting veterans from the narcissistic injuries of daily life on the home front. In terms echoed by other practitioners, McNally and Frueh (2013) describe the conditions for a dignified disability status:

> It is surely better to obtain disability payments for injuries, psychological as well as physical, sustained as a warrior than to receive welfare. Indeed, from being a valued member of a highly trained, professional armed forces unit, to being another nameless member of the unemployable segment of America's rejected class is a very difficult transition. Shame motivates righteous anger and steps to restore one's pride.
>
> (p. 525)

Evaluators experience some of these anxieties over protecting the psychic armor of veterans and their loss of special status after military service. The PTSD diagnosis provides sufficient flexibility at the symptom level to cover a wide range of these "narcissistic injuries" while grounding the complaints in a traumatic stressor that can be as elusive to verify as it is concrete in its narrative specificity.

Morel (1998) developed his own scale, the Morel Emotional Numbing Test (MENT), which he recommends for differential diagnosis of PTSD, as well as for separating genuine from factitious cases. Although the PTSD trauma script requires a dramatic life-threatening story, accompanied by severe symptoms, evaluators caution that "overly dramatic" accounts are common indicators of malingering or factitious PTSD. While a key area of symptomatology involves difficulties in affect regulation, post-deployment states of emotional lability—of extreme mood swings—are quite common and can be difficult to distinguish clinically from PTSD (Frueh, Hamner, Cahill, Gold, & Hamlin, 2000; McNally, 2003; Resnick, 2003). The Catch-22 for the plaintiff—and for the evaluator—centers on this seeming paradox. The threshold for believability requires that the story establish the externality of the cause without the air of a grievance against the military itself.

PTSD complaints carry some element of what psychoanalysis terms *transference*—experiencing a powerful authority figure in the present as though they were someone in the past. It's easier to go after the VA than the commander that put you in harm's way. As I suggested in taking up the case of John King in the first chapter, military commanders, many of whom foster childhood transferences as the "good father," are now nowhere around. The soldier's story of PTSD permits accounts of violent confrontations, specifically at the hands of the enemy, but offers little validation for child-like feelings of emotional abandonment. Losing your buddy is an authorized stress. But losing daddy is not.

Where there is transference, there is also countertransference. Clinicians bring their own unconscious conflicts and identifications to their encounters with veterans, as do veterans seeking care. Class prejudices and stereotypes infuse countertransference reactions, whether in romanticizing combat veterans as "war heroes" or in casting veterans who exaggerate symptoms as losers. Although insightful and compassionate in his descriptions of disability claimants, Resnick (2003) adopts a more dismissive tone in describing veterans suspected of malingering: "Malingerers are more likely to be marginal members of society with few binding ties or committed long-standing financial responsibilities, such as home ownership" (pp. 192–193). The focus on home ownership expresses a notable middle-class sensibility for what counts as binding commitments.

Munchausen syndrome holds a close affinity with cases of exaggerated PTSD symptoms (Resnick, 2003). The two conditions also bring storytelling to the center of the diagnostic process. British psychiatrist Michael Baggaley (1998) presents data from a psychiatric center in the UK where reviewers found that 13 percent of patients seeking care for PTSD over a period of a year were proved to be factitious (the term for conditions that are faked in order to solicit medical attention). In his report on "Military Munchausen's," Baggaley notes that veterans commonly report dramatic battle scenes that are unlikely to have occurred. He introduces two categories of false reporting: those with no prior military experience and those who served but make false claims about their involvement in operations. Baggaley notes that it is easier to detect those who have never served, particularly for clinicians with military experience. If a patient begins by claiming, "I've been in the SAS," it is worth noting the number of books and films on the Special Air Service and the romantic appeal of these forces for many young men. Patients may explain in hushed tones that they were part of a secret operation—a ruse employed to stitch over gaps in the story as classified information. Also suspicious are highly dramatic or elaborate war stories that seem scripted or told without much affect.

Obscured in Baggaley's tips for detecting deception are the interactive dynamics of clinical assessment encounters. Oddly, the reference to Military Munchausen's in the article's title is not taken up directly in the paper itself. Described in great detail elsewhere in the psychiatric literature, the condition was named after Baron Munchausen, a character in an 18th-century German novel written by Rudolf Erich Raspe. The character travelled widely, inventing stories that captivated others. The syndrome, identified by British physician Richard Asher in 1951, registered the close and intertwined histories of the military and medicine. Baron Munchausen, having served in the Prussian army, was reputed to entertain people with his tall tales of ventures abroad. The psychiatric syndrome referred to people who produce elaborate stories, often accompanied by self-inflicted symptoms, for the purposes of securing medical care. Doctors would perform unnecessary surgeries or medical procedures because the patients were so effective in presenting symptoms associated with known illnesses. These patients had been variously labeled as hysterics, hypochondriacs, and fakers.

But Munchausen syndrome carried a certain dignity and element of compassion that distinguished it from other diagnoses associated with faking illness. The patient was understood to be hungrily seeking attention, cleverly deceiving their doctors and entangling them in endless consultations—but suffering from a mental infirmity not of their own making. Asher (1951) brought into medical discourse a keen awareness of the non-rational and unconscious aspects of the diagnostic process, with Munchausen syndrome serving as prototype: "Like the famous Baron von Munchausen, the persons affected have always travelled widely; and their stories, like those attributed to him, are both dramatic and untruthful. Accordingly, the syndrome is respectfully dedicated to the Baron, and named after him" (p. 339). While the clinical literature focuses on signs of the disorder, Asher's description spoke to emotional reactions on the part of clinicians, including anxieties in the medical profession over being "manipulated" by a patient. Munchausen syndrome is as much a condition of the medical profession as it is of patients, however, in registering the role of captivating stories in clinical care.

Later named factitious disorder, a condition where the patient creates symptoms for the purpose of securing medical treatment, Munchausen syndrome still circulates in hospital hallway consultations among doctors. For the VA system, including disability payment system, Munchausen-like cases exceed available sorting instruments. It may be easier to separate fakers from the truly disabled than to work with the many veterans that do not conform to either of these starkly limited prototypes. And returning soldiers do often sense that that they are evaluated on the basis of the evocative power of their war stories. As a result, PTSD may be the most readily available container for diffuse sources of distress among veterans, many of whom do look to a VA Castle on the hill for some relief from less readily articulated miseries of military service and the return home.

Variants of PTSD have generated considerable controversy, particularly as feminists have attempted to fit women's grievances into the Procrustean bed of DSM nosology. Ralph Slovenko (2003) describes the challenges of forensic experts called to explain how rape trauma syndrome and battered women syndrome conform to the standard picture for posttraumatic stress disorder. Daniel Shuman (1995) claims that because DSM criteria does not distinguish these sub-types, "a cottage industry of experts has developed to offer their services to litigants on these distinctions" (p. 5). He describes a shift in the legal system in the United States over the past half century from reliance on lay witness testimony to expert testimony.

## Disabling Female Grievances

Squaring off on the politics of VA disability benefits for PTSD, defenders and critics each carry an important truth. Defenders of veterans' claims stress the history of denial by the Department of Defense concerning the long-term psychological consequences of warfare. In assigning the VA with this postwar work, the DoD is able to institutionally repress these effects and to keep the consequences of their own military missions out of sight. The long-term institutional burdens of warfare fall hardest on the VA system, which tends to secure less funding and certainly less glory than the DoD and its Armed Forces. Yet critics counter that the VA has nurtured a culture of disability and that evaluators are the enablers of this pathogenic system (Gade, 2013). The broader contexts influencing disability claims—and how the system serves as a portal for more diffuse grievances of veterans—are readily obscured in this either/or dichotomous framing of the issues.

The disability system within the VA does recognize the special entitlements of veterans. Unlike workers compensation or civil cases, VA procedures are written with the aim of making them non-adversarial (Worthen & Moering, 2011). The government is required to assist the veteran in preparing the case, including in securing relevant records. The examiner must determine that the disability was "at least as likely as not" (50 percent or greater) caused by the stressor event, as opposed to the legal standard of "preponderance of the evidence" (greater than 50 percent). These highly subjective judgment calls reflect a value in the system that signals to the examiners that the benefit of doubt should tilt in the direction of the veteran. Yet this very ethos of care, much like the imago of the "good mother," sets the stage for bitter disappointment when it fails to deliver on its promise of nurture.

Women warriors, however, *are* routinely left behind in military culture. The PTSD movement of the 1970s grew out of solidarity between veterans and feminists around the issue of trauma and violence. But the sexual division of storytelling around disability claims establishes a very high bar for women veterans in advancing their complaints. Although female service members score higher than males on measures of PTSD, women are less likely to receive disability benefits. Historically, combat exposure was one of the leading criteria for service-related trauma exposure (Murdoch et al., 2003). Since women were barred until 2013 from combat roles in the US armed services, they faced a higher threshold in documenting claims for service-related disabilities. Women veterans, relative to their male counterparts, are more likely to be poor and to lack access to healthcare. The stories of impoverished female veterans are less apt to move assessors than those of their male comrades within a larger VA culture less receptive to their needs.

In 2013 and shortly before the drawdown of United States forces in Afghanistan, the Department of Defense rescinded the Direct Combat Exclusion Rule on women serving in restricted military occupation. For many feminists, overturning discriminatory barriers to combat and the elite Special Forces represented a highly prized marker of progress. While women had served in combat roles in many countries for some time, the question of whether female participation in the dirtiest business of war—direct combat and the psychological changes that accompany that training—had since the Vietnam War generated heated debate in the United States. Feminist critiques of patriarchy often centered on unpacking and dismantling the culture of warfare. Yet military service had its benefits. Combat represented the lethal borders of that service where the risks were greatest. But so too were the rewards. Since President Obama declared the long wars were close to conclusion, public anxiety was abated over women joining the highly masculinized brotherhood of the infantry. After all, women were entering the battlefield as the brigades were returning home.

Political focus on women in the military had reached a fever pitch during those same years, however, around a new wave of cases of sexual assault related to disability claims. The Ruth Moore Act of 2013 in the United States Congress was in response to public concerns over the treatment of female veterans filing disability claims based on military sexual trauma (MST). MST includes a wide spectrum of misconduct, from persistent unwanted attention and disparaging comments to rape and having sex when too drunk to consent. The act was named in honor of a Navy sailor who fought the VA for decades to secure disability benefits based on a diagnosis of PTSD and her history of military sexual trauma. Moore reported having been raped twice by her supervisor shortly after joining the Navy and repeatedly having claims rejected after developing mental health problems. Although VA data conclude that half of MST survivors are men, the rates are overall higher among female service members since women comprise only 14% of the Armed Forces. Female veterans and their advocates pushed Congress through the Ruth Moore Act to change standards of proof to allow more weight to the veteran's story in cases of MST, arguing that barriers within the military made documentation of sexual assault extremely difficult. The bill extended a trend already underway in PTSD disability claims to rely less on official military records in evaluating claims and to give more weight to clinical assessments. But female veterans continued to confront barriers. Benefits for PTSD overwhelmingly favored male veterans with service-related stressors and denied the majority of PTSD claims by female service members. The explanation for rejected claims tended to cite the lack of adequate documentation.

A widely distributed study by Yale Veterans Legal Services, published in 2013 by the ACLU and the Service Women's Action Network, concluded that nearly 16,000 veterans made MST-related PTSD disability benefit claims during the five-year period of the study, 66.1 percent of whom were female veterans. Male veterans making claims based on MST-related PTSD were more likely to have their claims denied than were female veterans (Veterans Legal Services Clinic, Yale Law School, 2013). But there were also far fewer of them. Because women's PTSD disability claims were more apt to be based on military sexual trauma than hostile fire, the report argued that VA protocols were inherently discriminatory against female service members.

Yet even with the passage of the Ruth Moore Act, subsequent reports have documented this persisting bias. The Servicemembers and Veterans Empowerment and Support Act was introduced in the 2019–2020 session of Congress and argues that further changes in the law are necessary to push the VA to take more seriously this discriminatory bias. The Department of Veterans Services pushed back against this further liberalization of the law (Gross, 2019).

The heated controversy over gender biases in disability claims carries a strong echo of the early PTSD movement when feminists and anti-war activists argued for combat and rape as the prototypes for societally produced trauma. As MST emerged on the frontlines of what the ACLU termed the "Battle for Benefits," this fight for the rights of female veterans centered on post-war grievances, just as male veterans had fought the government for various rights and benefits after previous wars. Unlike exposure to hostile fire, however, MST cases implicated military institutions in the troubles of warfare in a more intimate way.

The Veterans Health Administration authorized counseling for sexual assault in the early 1990s, and MST services became a permanent benefit by 2004, along with required screening for sexual trauma and designated coordinators at all VA regional centers to oversee MST treatment and training. As recruitment for the wars in Afghanistan and Iraq expanded, the military shift to projecting a more caring ethos extended to displaying more sensitivity to female service members. While MST topped the list of service-related risks for female recruits, therapists played leading roles in framing links between the responses of female veterans to the new critical items on post-deployment screenings and the range of troubles these same veterans reported at VA clinics. A vast army of therapists emerged to assist women in creating a compelling clinical picture.

At a 2013 Pacific Northwest conference on military sexual trauma that I attended, the role of clinicians in framing the condition was very much on display, including in responses to VA handling of disability claims. The opening session of the conference offered dramatic readings based on the experiences of veterans—titled "MST Monologues." The monologues were written by veterans of different eras of military conflict—four women and one man—and read by conference speakers. The stories carried the distinctive markers of therapeutic culture. They were structured around the trauma/betrayal model—an approach that explains trauma as a result of ruptures in the sense of basic trust in the world. One of the guiding principles of the model is that traumatic violations of trust produce forms of dissociation—feelings of emotional detachment or numbing—and can include amnesia for the traumatic event itself. Therapists routinely enlist the concept of body memory to explain how physical and/or psychiatric symptoms fortify this amnesiac protective barrier by protecting consciousness from the pain of recollecting a traumatic event. Later in life, the amnesiac barrier may rupture and allow the memory to break through into consciousness. While context does influence recall and memory retrieval, social contexts can also stimulate mental images that feel memory-like. While dissociative reactions are indeed common effects of trauma, less readily acknowledged by trauma specialists is the role of thera-pists in structuring memory retrieval and the creation of a coherent narrative (Haaken, 1998).

The first monologue, authored by an Operation New Dawn veteran (the war in Afghanistan), begins with her decision to enlist after the Septem-ber 11 attacks on the World Trade Center. She was not involved in combat but did serve in zones of firefights—one of the traditional qualifiers for dis-ability claims. A fellow Marine pursues her, although she doesn't explain what actually happened. Her story focuses on the destructive aftermath of a sexual assault and her years of disturbing symptoms: self-blame, drinking heavily, and cutting herself. Her feelings of betrayal focus on the military command structure and on the injustice of being charged under Article 18 with malingering. She concludes by saying that her therapist thought she had a good basis for a claim and that she is now on disability for PTSD and depression.

One of the more dramatic monologues was authored by a male veteran who had been in the Marine Corps in Vietnam. The story starts with his grief as a teenager after losing his mother to suicide. He then ran away from home to join the Marine Corp, which became his supportive substitute family. Dec-ades after serving and after having a family of his own, he recalls a horrifying night during his deployment in Vietnam. The brutal scene at the center of the memory involved a commander and his wife coercing him into a series of sexual games after inviting him to their home for dinner. The sex games esca-lated and culminated with the commander raping him while his wife looked on. The monologue concludes with the Marine explaining how this recollection of military sexual trauma gave him the courage and conviction to go forward with a disability claim.

The next monologue, authored by a World War II female veteran, was intro-duced by the speaker to illustrate the intergenerational and longstanding nature of PTSD and how this was a problem during the "good war" as well as in more recent military conflicts. She describes serving in the Pacific theater and initially feeling valued for her contribution to the war effort, heightened by a wondrous sense of adventure. She recalls being good-looking but also a good girl—sexually chaste—with a fiancé back home. There was an initial feeling of safety in serving the US military before her sense of security was shattered. One evening after leaving the mess hall, a fellow soldier ripped off her clothes and molested her while she was walking back to her barracks. She describes the violence of the attack as well as the rupture of her state of mind. In the early 2000s, she visits a VA doctor who asks her if she had been sexually assaulted during her service in the military. Initially downplaying the significance of the event, she recalls that her perpetrator had called her a dirty whore. On the recommendation of her doctor, she starts therapy for PTSD, feeling that the trauma of that event had made her avoid contact with people and had created distance even with her own children. She testifies to the possibilities for healing from trauma even as an elderly person and how therapy helped her to regain some of what had been stolen from her that dark night on the Pacific Front.

Whether or not these events occurred as remembered, the military sexual trauma story came onto the public stage as the one testimonial where veterans could be seen and heard. Indeed, it was codified by the military as a risk for female service members and part of the package of veterans' benefits. Cultural scripts offer narrative materials for clinicians as they assist in this process, however. One of these scripts centers on the female protagonist's loss of innocence through a journey beyond the protective confines of familial safety. Whereas journeys of passage for male protagonists include various tests of manhood, many of the traditional stories available to female protagonists create drama around the dangers of exploratory freedom and the loss of moral and sexual purity.

As women, there is a certain allowance in these accounts to express outrage against the command structure for its failures to protect female warriors and to give voice to the sexually abusive aspects of military culture. Whereas male veterans may narrate their PTSD stories around a loss of innocence, the rupture tends to center on shattered illusions of invulnerability. The MST narratives mobilize public sympathies through a similar loss of innocence but within a very narrow field of military experiences. The admixture of sexual desire and violation, of a larger struggle with military culture or moral questioning of the war missions, are not readily integrated into the MST narrative. Support for the account—particularly as a disability claim—depends heavily on the emotional skills of the storyteller and her ability to establish a condition of absolute innocence and ruination. Narratively, the testimonies are melodramas structured around a familial struggle and starkly drawn virtuous and villainous characters. The expansion of MST as the leading category for female disability claims signifies progress but at a considerable cost for female veterans. Therapists enlisted in assessing these cases may reproduce traditional notions of being "damaged goods" and that disability itself is a marker of a violated virtuous woman (Haaken, 2016).

## Conclusions

The PTSD movement grew out of opposition to the Vietnam War and brought mental disabilities to the center of veterans' war stories. Veterans' rights groups organized to liberalize criteria for compensation based on the PTSD diagnosis, although winning a claim increasingly relies on psychiatric expertise rather than on the military record or the veteran's story of military service. The trauma story is important, but the main storytelling centers on the nexus of causal connections between a past event and the disabling symptoms in the present. The PTSD diagnosis bars the complex histories that contribute to the current clinical picture, including conflicts with the military itself. It may be easier to sign off on disability claims than to listen to the many distressing accounts of veterans—or to explore the ambiguous psychological and social terrain of so many disability cases. To declare a veteran disabled is to confer recognition for a claim on society for support. But the diagnosis can itself be disabling as a pronouncement by an expert, and particularly when the alternative judgments are "fakers" and "malingerers." PSTD offers a dignified path of dependency on social welfare services for veterans—one that maintains defensive distance from the fates of other marginalized groups subject to the harsh stigma and punitive policies of the American welfare state.

For female veterans, the gender dynamics around disability claims confront a quite different set of obstacles. MST brings the pathology of military culture into the PTSD narrative but within a narrow relational field. Congressional support across the political divide for liberalizing MST-based disability claims in the 21st century has depended heavily on clinical reports that domesticate female veterans' complaints. Within the MST literature, commanders who either abuse women under their command or look the other way when abuse occurs in their ranks tend to be framed as failed father figures. But the military is not a family, as so many service members find after completing their tours of duty. Actual fathers who describe their jobs as getting the most of their children as "assets"— who approach fatherhood in such an instrumental way—would most certainly be judged sociopathic. Good commanders understand their duties to protect their troops and the importance of inspiring genuine trust and respect. But they also understand that relationships within their unit are driven by military missions.

The final chapter brings more of the social psychology of trauma diagnoses into the picture by looking at groups of users—communities of sufferers— that have embraced, accepted, or resisted the PTSD diagnosis. The lessons include cautionary tales on the application of psychiatric expertise in situations where people are struggling for recognition, while dependent on a system that excludes their suffering from the psychiatric field of vision.

## References

American Psychiatric Association. (2013). *Diagnostic and statistical manual of mental disorders (DSM-5)*. Washington, DC: Author.

Asch, S. M., McGlynn, E. A., Hogan, M. M., Hayward, R. A., Shekelle, P., Rubenstein, L., . . . Kerr, E. A. (2004). Comparison of quality of care for patients in the Veterans

Health Administration and patients in a national sample. *Annals of Internal Medicine*, *141*(12), 938-W-213.

Asher, R. (1951). Munchausen's syndrome. *The Lancet*, *257*(6650), 339–341.

Baggaley, M. (1998). "Military Munchausen's": Assessment of factitious claims of military service in psychiatric patients. *Psychiatric Bulletin*, *22*(3), 153–154. https://doi.org/10.1192/pb.22.3.153

Bernton, H. (2012b, February 7). Madigan memo on PTSD costs sparked Army review. *The Seattle Times*. Retrieved from www.seattletimes.com/seattle-news/madigan-memo-on-ptsd-costs-sparked-army-review/

Bernton, H. (2012a, March 20). 40% of PTSD diagnoses at Madigan were reversed. *The Seattle Times*. Retrieved from www.seattletimes.com/seattle-news/40-of-ptsd-diagnoses-at-madigan-were-reversed/

Blanchfield, L., & Brown, C. (2015). *The United Nations convention on the rights of persons with disabilities: Issues in the U.S. ratification debate* (No. CRS Report R42749). Retrieved from Congressional Research Service website: https://fas.org/sgp/crs/misc/R42749.pdf

Brewin, C. R., Lanius, R. A., Novac, A., Schnyder, U., & Galea, S. (2009). Reformulating PTSD for DSM-V: Life after Criterion A. *Journal of Traumatic Stress*, *22*(5), 366–373. https://doi.org/10.1002/jts.20443

Brown, W. B. (2008). Another emerging "storm": Iraq and Afghanistan veterans with PTSD in the criminal justice system. *Justice Policy Journal*, *5*(2), 1–37.

Bryan, C. J., & Morrow, C. E. (2011). Circumventing mental health stigma by embracing the warrior culture: Lessons learned from the defender's edge program. *Professional Psychology—Research & Practice February 2011*, *42*(1), 16–23. https://doi.org/10.1037/a0022290

Calandrillo, S. P. (2006). *An economic analysis of the eggshell plaintiff rule* (Working Paper No. 19). Retrieved from The Berkeley Electronic Press website: https://law.bepress.com/cgi/viewcontent.cgi?referer=www.google.com/&httpsredir=1&article=1830&context=alea

Charcot, J.-M. (1888). *Clinical lectures on certain diseases of the nervous system* (E. P. Hurt, Trans.). Philadelphia, PA: Davis.

Crabb, T., & Segal, D. R. (2018). Comparative systems of analysis: Military sociology in the United States and Europe. In G. Caforio & M. Nuciari (Eds.), *Handbook of the sociology of the military* (2nd ed., pp. 61–86). New York, NY: Springer.

Crosby, C. (2017, April 19). *Tinnitus, the most claimed disability in the VA* [Blog post]. Retrieved from Hill & Ponton Disability Attorneys website: www.hillandponton.com/tinnitus-claimed-disability-va/

Dickson, P., & Allen, T. B. (2006). *The Bonus Army: An American epic*. New York, NY: Walker Books.

Erichsen, J. E. (1867). *On railway and other injuries of the nervous system*. Philadelphia, PA: Henry C. Lea.

Fagelson, M. A. (2007). The association between tinnitus and posttraumatic stress disorder. *American Journal of Audiology*, *16*(2), 107–117. https://doi.org/10.1044/1059-0889(2007/015)

Fairbairn, W. R. D. (1943). The war neuroses: Their nature and significance. *The British Medical Journal*, *1*(4284), 183–186. Retrieved from www.jstor.org/stable/20325356

Frueh, B. C., Grubaugh, A. L., Elhai, J. D., & Buckley, T. C. (2007). US Department of Veterans Affairs disability policies for posttraumatic stress disorder: Administrative trends and implications for treatment, rehabilitation, and research. *American Journal of Public Health, 97*(12), 2143–2145. https://doi.org/10.2105/AJPH.2007.115436

Frueh, B. C., Hamner, M. B., Cahill, S. P., Gold, P. B., & Hamlin, K. L. (2000). Apparent symptom overreporting in combat veterans evaluated for PTSD. *Clinical Psychology Review, 20*(7), 853–885. https://doi.org/10.1016/S0272-7358(99)00015-X

Gade, D. M. (2013). A better way to help veterans. *National Affairs, 41*(Summer). Retrieved from www.nationalaffairs.com/publications/detail/a-better-way-to-help-veterans

Gold, L. H. (2003). PTSD in employment litigation. In R. I. Simon (Ed.), *Posttraumatic stress disorder in litigation: Guidelines for forensic assessment* (2nd ed., pp. 163–186). Arlington, VA: American Psychiatric Publishing, Inc.

Green, B. L., & Kaltman, S. I. (2003). Recent research findings on the diagnosis of PTSD: Prevalence, course, comorbidity, and risk. In R. I. Simon (Ed.), *Posttraumatic stress disorder in litigation: Guidelines for forensic assessment* (2nd ed., pp. 19–39). Arlington, VA: American Psychiatric Association.

Green, D. (2016, August 12). *Taking care of our heroes, because they took care of us.* Retrieved March 26, 2019, from Vantage Point website: www.blogs.va.gov/VAntage/30048/taking-care-of-veterans/

Gross, N. (2019, June 21). *How far should victims have to go to prove military sexual trauma?* Retrieved February 21, from *Military Times.* Website: www.militarytimes.com/news/pentagon-congress/2019/06/21/how-far-should-victims-have-to-go-to-prove-military-sexual-trauma

Haaken, J. (1998). *Pillar of salt: Gender, memory, and the perils of looking back.* New Brunswick, NJ: Rutgers University Press.

Haaken, J. (2012). Picturing the field: Social action research, psychoanalytic theory and documentary filmmaking. In P. Reavey (Ed.), *Visual methods in psychology* (pp. 223–240). New York, NY: Routledge.

Haaken, J. (2014). *Mind zone: Therapists behind the front lines* [Documentary]. United States: Herzog & Company.

Haaken, J. (2016). Riding the waves of feminism: Psychoanalysis and women's liberation. *Psychoanalysis, Culture & Society, 21*(3), 223–231. https://doi.org/10.1057/pcs.2016.5

Haaken, J., & O'Neill, M. (2014). Keepin' it real: Social action research, psychoanalytic theory, and the moving to the beat project. In B. Roberts & A. Sparkes (Eds.), *Advances in biographical methods* (pp. 43–54). London, UK: Palgrave Macmillan. https://doi.org/10.4324/9781315851372-11

Harbaugh, K. (2017, December 21). The risk of over-thanking our veterans. *The New York Times.* Retrieved from www.nytimes.com/2015/06/01/opinion/the-risk-of-over-thanking-our-veterans.html

Higonnet, M. R. (1987). *Behind the lines: Gender and the two World Wars.* New Haven, CT: Yale University Press.

Higonnet, M. R., & Higonnet, P. (1987). The double helix. In M. R. Higonnet, J. Jenson, S. Michel, & M. C. Weitz (Eds.), *Reading behind the lines. Postmemory in contemporary British war fiction* (pp. 31–47). New Haven, CT: Yale University Press.

Koch, W. J., Douglas, K. S., Nicholls, T. L., & O'Neill, M. L. (2006). *Psychological injuries: Forensic assessment, treatment, and law* (R. Roesch, Ed.). New York, NY: Oxford University Press.

Lembcke, J. (1998). The "right stuff" gone wrong: Vietnam veterans and the social construction of post-traumatic stress disorder. *Critical Sociology, 24*(1/2), 37–64. https://doi.org/10.1177/089692059802400104

Levy, M. I. (1995, November). Stressing the point: When are post traumatic stress claims legitimate . . . and when are they not? *For the Defense.* Retrieved from www.experts.com/Articles/Post-Traumatic-Stress-Disorder-Claim-By-Mark-Levy

Loughran, T. (2009). Shell-Shock and psychological medicine in First World War Britain. *Social History of Medicine, 22*(1), 79–95. https://doi.org/10.1093/shm/hkn093

MacGregor, C., & Heilemann, M. V. (2017). Deserving veterans' disability compensation: A qualitative study of veterans' perceptions. *Health & Social Work, 42*(2), e86–e93. https://doi.org/10.1093/hsw/hlx017

McDougall, J. (1974). The psychosoma and the psychoanalytic process. *International Review of Psycho-Analysis, 1,* 437–459.

McNally, R. J. (2003). Progress and controversy in the study of posttraumatic stress disorder. *Annual Review of Psychology, 54,* 229–252. https://doi.org/10.1146/annurev.psych.54.101601.145112

McNally, R. J., & Frueh, B. C. (2013). Why are Iraq and Afghanistan War veterans seeking PTSD disability compensation at unprecedented rates? *Journal of Anxiety Disorders, 27*(5), 520–526. https://doi.org/10.1016/j.janxdis.2013.07.002

McQuade, J. S. (2001). The eggshell skull rule and related problems in recovery for mental harm in the Law of Torts. *Campbell Law Review, 24*(1), 1–45.

Mittelstadt, J. (2015). *The rise of the military welfare state.* Cambridge, MA: Harvard University Press.

Montopoli, B. (2012, December 4). *U.N. treaty on disabilities falls short in Senate.* Retrieved from CBS News website: www.cbsnews.com/news/un-treaty-on-disabilities-falls-short-in-senate/

Morel, K. R. (1998). Development and preliminary validation of a forced-choice test of response bias for posttraumatic stress disorder. *Journal of Personality Assessment, 70*(2), 299–314. https://doi.org/10.1207/s15327752jpa7002_8

Morel, K. R. (2010). *Differential diagnosis of malingering versus posttraumatic stress disorder: Scientific rationale and objective scientific methods.* Hauppauge, N.Y: Nova Science Publishers, Inc.

Murdoch, M., Hodges, J., Hunt, C., Cowper, D., Kressin, N., & O'Brien, N. (2003). Gender differences in service connection for PTSD. *Medical Care, 41*(8), 950–961.

Murphy, K. (2012, February 21). Army avoiding PTSD claims? Madigan chief suspended amid inquiry. *Los Angeles Times.* Retrieved from http://articles.latimes.com/2012/feb/21/nation/la-na-nn-ptsd-army-madigan-20120221

Nash, W. P., & Litz, B. T. (2013). Moral injury: A mechanism for war-related psychological trauma in military family members. *Clinical Child and Family Psychology Review, 16*(4), 365–375.

Ozner, E. J., & Weiss, D. S. (2004). Who develops posttraumatic stress disorder? *Current Directions in Psychological Science, 13*(4), 169–172. https://doi.org/10.2307/20182942

Phillips, A. (2014). *Becoming Freud: The making of a psychoanalyst.* Yale University Press.

Prestwich, P. E. (2003). "Victims of war"? Mentally-traumatized soldiers and the state, 1918–1939. *Journal of the Western Society for French History*, *31*, 243–254.

Resnick, P. J. (2003). Guidelines for evaluation of malingering patients in PTSD. In R. I. Simon (Ed.), *Posttraumatic stress disorder in litigation: Guidelines for forensic assessment* (2nd ed., pp. 187–205). Arlington, VA: American Psychiatric Publishing.

Ruiz, R. (2013, March 15). Army releases findings of Madigan PTSD investigation. *NBC News*. Retrieved from http://usnews.nbcnews.com/_news/2013/03/15/17330146-army-releases-findings-of-madigan-ptsd-investigation

Schivelbusch, W. (1979). *The railway journey: Trains and travel in the 19th century*. New York, NY: Urizen Books.

Scioli, E. R., Otis, J. D., & Keane, T. M. (2010). Psychological problems associated with Operation Enduring Freedom/Operation Iraqi Freedom deployment. *American Journal of Lifestyle Medicine*, *4*(4), 349–359.

Shay, J. (2003). *Odysseus in America: Combat trauma and the trials of homecoming*. New York, NY: Simon and Schuster.

Shay, J. (2014). Moral injury. *Psychoanalytic Psychology*, *31*(2), 182–191. https://doi.org/10.1037/a0036090

Shulkin, D., & Sheetz, K. (2019, January 6). Reforming veterans benefits will be controversial, but necessary. *The Hill*. Retrieved from https://thehill.com/opinion/white-house/424037-reforming-veterans-benefits-will-be-controversial-but-necessary

Shuman, D. (1995). Persistent reexperiences in psychiatry and law: Current and future trends for the role of PTSD in litigation. In R. I. Simon (Ed.), *Posttraumatic stress disorder in litigation: Guidelines for forensic assessment* (pp. 1–18). Arlington, VA: American Psychiatric Association.

Slovenko, R. (2003). Introduction. In R. I. Simon (Ed.), *Posttraumatic stress disorder in litigation: Guidelines for forensic assessment* (2nd ed., p. 24). Arlington, VA: American Psychiatric Association.

Stone, A. A. (1993). Post-traumatic stress disorder and the law: Critical review of the new frontier. *Journal of the American Academy of Psychiatry and the Law Online*, *21*(1), 23–36

van der Kolk, B. A. (2002). Posttraumatic therapy in the age of neuroscience. *Psychoanalytic Dialogues*, *12*(3), 381–392. https://doi.org/10.1080/10481881209348674

Veterans Legal Services Clinic, Yale Law School. (2013). *The battle for benefits report*. Retrieved from www.aclu.org/battle-benefits-va-discrimination-against-survivors-military-sexual-trauma

Wadsworth, M. (n.d.). *How to apply for veterans disability benefits*. Retrieved May 1, 2019, from Nolo website: www.nolo.com/legal-encyclopedia/how-apply-veterans-disability-benefits.html

Wagner, B. (2009). Kafka's office writings: Historical background and institutional setting. In *Franz Kafka: The office writings* (pp. 19–50). Princeton, NJ: Princeton University Press.

Wessely, S. (2005). War stories: Invited commentary on . . . documented combat exposure of US veterans seeking treatment for combat-related post-traumatic stress disorder. *The British Journal of Psychiatry, 186*(6), 473–475. https://doi.org/10.1192/bjp.186.6.473

Wilson, E. (2010, July 12). VA eases claims process for veterans with PTSD. *Department of Defense News.* Retrieved from www.defense.gov/news/newsarticle.aspx?id=59987

Worthen, M. D., & Moering, R. G. (2011). A practical guide to conducting VA compensation and pension exams for PTSD and other mental disorders. *Psychological Injury and Law, 4*(3–4), 187–216. https://doi.org/10.1007/s12207-011-9115-2

Yardley, W. (2012, March 11). Killings add to worries at Joint Base Lewis-McChord. *The New York Times.* Retrieved from www.nytimes.com/2012/03/12/us/killings-add-to-worries-at-joint-base-lewis-mcchord.html

Zarembo, A. (2014, July 12). With U.S. encouragement, VA disability claims rise sharply. *Los Angeles Times.* Retrieved from www.latimes.com/local/la-me-veterans-disability-20140713-story.html

# Chapter 5

# Suffering Together

## Group Responses to Trauma

In carrying out field projects in England, West Africa, and the United States, I became interested in how collective accounts of suffering migrate across national borders and acquire socially symbolic currency in the process. By socially symbolic, I mean that the factual basis of the story may become less important over time than its mythic truth—its capacity to transcend the concrete circumstances of suffering. Stories change in the telling and retelling of them, adapting to local customs (Bruner & Lucariello, 1989; Kintsch & Greene, 1978). Effective transmitters of tales must develop an attunement to what local listeners are able or willing to hear.

Good listening skills—listening with a "third ear"—depend on understanding cultural filters for believability. In interviewing refugees that fled the Sierra Leonean civil war in the late 1990s, a number of the women described the horrors they had endured when rebels overtook their villages (Haaken, Ladum, Tarr, Zundel, & Heymann, 2005). One account strained my personal believability filters, even as it pressed me to think further about what makes a story feel true. Several women told of teenage soldiers with the Revolutionary United Front who would routinely cut open pregnant women and rip out their fetuses and then proceed to cook and eat them. The stories included reports of these soldiers raping their own mothers. Yet no one had actually seen these events. They were stories passed on as rumors, although there was evidence that killing, amputating villagers' limbs, and rapes were part of the terrorist arsenal of the rebels. Over time, I came to understand these elaborations as attempts to break through a wall of colonial indifference to their suffering. While some psychiatric readings might view the accounts as expressions of group hysteria, I came to view them as expressions of extreme distress.

As socially symbolic narratives, the stories captured the agonizing poetics of the tragedy. The rebel war ripped open the very heart and soul of the country. As I became known by Sierra Leonean youth as Mama Jan, I also became attuned to how older women are commonly addressed as "mama," and to the flexibility of maternal categories in the matrilineal kinship structures of this region of Africa. So "raping your mother" extended across a wide terrain of Sierra Leonean society. The *rebel war*—as it was often called—was different from so many civil wars in that the rebels attacked their own villages rather than a cultural group marked as outsiders or the "Other." Some of the grievances of these alienated youth centered on a patriarchal system where young men were cut off from the resources of their village, with heavy fines levied for infractions, such as having sex with young women who were in arranged marriages to the older men. While the rebels may not have raped their biological mothers, many had returned to their home villages to destroy them—even firebombing the houses of elders. Just as rape may be used as a metaphor in describing environmental destruction, for example, in decrying the "rape of Mother Earth," the invoking of this incest taboo and the violence of rape conveyed this same moral condemnation of the young rebels.

This chapter navigates the social psychology of PTSD, and specifically how social movements and political grievances have shaped the production of PTSD stories. My interest is in recovering some of the progressive animus of the early posttraumatic stress movement and its call for enlarging social responsibility for politically produced suffering. I explain how factors at the societal level have shaped diagnostic storytelling in Western countries no less than in the global South. My social psychology draws on feminist psychoanalysis—an approach that attends to the role of fantasies, anxieties, and defenses in group life. I show how the PTSD constellation of symptoms narrows the field of observations in ways that obscure important elements of the picture. In developing this line of critique, I enlist another important concept in the psychoanalytic tradition: the idea that the psychological significance of the clinical picture is often located on the periphery of what is most readily noticed.

## PTSD Across Cultural Borders

During the late 1990s, when I worked with Sierra Leonean women on the documentary *Diamonds, Guns, and Rice* (Haaken & Heymann, 2005), international women's organizations had won recognition of rape in the criminal courts. Rape was now listed as a war crime. As modern warfare generated higher rates of casualties among civilian populations than among combatants, images of female war victims increasingly appeared on the global stage. Rape, an instrument of war throughout much of history, took on a new iconographic power.

In the course of that documentary project, women frequently spoke of gender violence—a term that had gained currency, often as a euphemism for rape, in international aid organizations. When I visited a refugee camp in Guinea near the Sierra Leonean border, women reported the number of cases of gender violence they had identified in the camps. Trauma was part of their language of suffering but only vaguely related to the criteria for PTSD. Trauma was more often invoked as a troubling memory that interfered with post-war reconciliation efforts. "We have to put the war behind us," one Sierra Leonean children's counselor exclaimed, "or the trauma will never leave you." Others cautioned that trauma was the result of premature forgetting, of "putting the war too quickly behind us" (Haaken et al., 2005). Posttraumatic stress disorder took hold in conflict zones in the decade that followed, invoked as signifier of the uncertainties that arise and hopes that experts can help achieve the "posttraumatic" return to normalcy.

In the late 20th and early 21st centuries, PTSD came to dominate international mental health policy and NGO-based post-conflict interventions (Breslau, 2004; Fassin & Rechtman, 2009). At the same time, the global mental health field has been the site of intense controversy over the PTSD diagnosis. Anthropological psychiatrist Arthur Kleinman (2012) introduced the term *idioms of distress* to describe the variability in cultural practices for communicating disturbing states, and he calls for caution in universalizing Western diagnoses such as PTSD. Others working on global mental health seize on PTSD, however, as a framework for advancing universal human rights (Kinzie et al., 1982; Mollica et al., 1992; Mollica, Wyshak, de Marneffe, Khuon, & Lavelle, 1987). Didier Fassin and Richard Rechtman (2009) describe the international ascendance of PTSD in the context of the growing field of humanitarian psychiatry and the expanded role of testimonials by psychologists and psychiatrists in conflict zones. The authors describe what they term the new "psycho-traumatology of exile," where asylum seekers in Europe increasingly depend on certificates issued by mental health professionals to support their claims.

Critics argue that the PTSD diagnosis obscures more than it reveals about the sources of suffering in conflict zones. Vanessa Pupavac (2004) describes international aid programs and how "trauma eclipsed hunger in the 1990s as the issue flagged by international aid agencies" (p. 149). Derek Summerfield (1999) goes further, claiming that "this is not just a conceptual issue, but an ethical one" (p. 1454). He advances one of the more trenchant critiques of PTSD as a form of psychiatric imperialism. By the late 1990s, identification of posttraumatic stress disorder in war zones had emerged as a top priority of humanitarian aid organizations, including UNICEF, WHO, European Community Humanitarian Office, and many nongovernmental organizations.

Summerfield (1999) describes PTSD as a "pseudo-condition"—an import brought into conflict zones by Western experts that obscures the political nature of these conflicts and marginalizes calls for other forms of support. He describes the expansion of the diagnosis and how since the early 1980s, "trauma projects have rapidly become attractive and even fashionable for Western donors" (p. 1451). In illustrating the oppressiveness of trauma aid, he draws on experiences working in Rwanda after the genocide. Summerfield describes the "stampede of humanitarian agencies" to the region, first in response to destitute Tutsi refugees, where aid workers described the phenomenon of mass psychological traumatization. The pressures to generate data in support of the cross-cultural validity and reliability of trauma scales tend to overwhelm other helping initiatives. The first step is often to establish baseline knowledge of trauma, for which there often is no equivalent local term. He offers a hypothetical story to illustrate the neo-colonial impulses and hubris of such efforts:

> It is instructive to transpose what happened in Rwanda to the Jewish Holocaust. A project, planned from afar and deploying foreign conceptual frame-works and practices, is mobilized in mid-1945 to come in to assist those who have just emerged alive from the concentration camps. The project leaders have often not worked in the area before, and perhaps do not know its history. The project is funded, say, for one year. In that time it hopes to tackle the "trauma" of the Holocaust for survivors, not just their personal losses but their sense of what was done to their people as a people. By so doing it also expects to reduce future mental problems, and the likelihood that they will turn from victims into perpetrators who embrace violence and war. Would not such a project seem grossly simplistic and presumptuous, and throw up ethical questions?
>
> (p. 1457)

The author goes on to question the validity of the PTSD diagnosis in the global North as well, pointing to its role in the medicalizing of emotional suffering and the meager yield of practical results from the vast expenditures in PTSD research on the part of the Veterans Administration and National Institute of Mental Health.

In *Culture of Trauma*, Joshua Breslau (2004) acknowledges the tremendous appeal of the PTSD concept for workers committed to addressing the social roots of suffering. But he argues that the diagnosis has served as scientific rationale for military and political interventions under the banner of medical science. He poses the question of why this disorder has generated far more interest than other mental health problems, such as depression or anxiety conditions. Erica James (2004) concurs, suggesting that "the discourse of trauma has been an organizing trope that has motivated new forms of technocratic practices designed to manage new categories of people within a social field" (p. 131). PTSD interventions enable clinicians to address human rights abuses while appearing not to take sides, in part because the disorder came to be recognized as an affliction of victims and perpetrators alike. In separating the symptoms from the political context of the traumatic event itself, the diagnosis offered the appearance of political neutrality.

Anthropological psychiatrist Donald Spence (2001) points out how trauma stories that migrate across global boundaries acquire currencies in situations where the struggle for recognition becomes a struggle for survival. As refugees find their way across the barricades imposed at borders, the granting of passage can depend on the power of the story. As Spence explains:

> Once a refugee speaker learns the impact of the refugee survivor's tale, once he/she learns that the story can silence any listener and make

him/her hunger for the speaker's next words, it is hard to give it up and to learn to show him/herself as less of a hero and more as an ordinary person. The person is tempted to tell the same story because its shock appeal can be literally breathtaking, and it can be a spellbinding experience to watch its effect on the listener.

(p. 26)

If we accept the premise that psychic trauma results from experiences that overwhelm capacities to make sense of disturbing events, the translators on the scene carry considerable authority in structuring the meaning of subjective responses to those events. Clinicians assume a key role in the treatment of trauma syndromes, both in diagnostic labeling and in co-constructing explanations for the symptoms of distress. Clinicians are not typically prepared, however, to incorporate the psychology of groups in their assessments of these same conditions, including their own positions within those groups.

In order to survive, all cultures generate practices for responding to death, loss, and emotional pain born of human bodily vulnerability and the inevitability of suffering. The concept of trauma came to be associated with unnecessary suffering—and suffering for which causes could be identified and interventions posed. Although PTSD has been embraced as a universal psycho-physiological condition, in practice the diagnosis circulates in highly politicized settings— what Fassin (2012) terms the *moral economy* of assistance. Psychic trauma has displaced violence as a signifier of suffering that calls for a response. One critical question taken up in the course of this book involves the role of diagnosticians in responding to that call.

## Feminism and Female Maladies

Dissociative identity disorder, termed multiple personality disorder (MPD) in the DSM-III, emerged as a hotly debated site of competing claims in the 1990s and was itself a response to the women's movement. Second-wave feminists of the 1970s were among the most ardent critics of psychiatric diagnoses and the DSM manuals. The rape survivor syndrome joined the Vietnam syndrome as conditions that were produced by societal forms of violence. Both women and veterans had for over a century been subject to the paranoid psychiatric gaze, scrutinized for signs of faking or malingering. The PTSD movement joined campaigns to "break the silence," to expose culturally repressed trauma, and to show how psychiatric expertise had been routinely enlisted to undermine the accounts of victims.

Multiple personality disorder, a disorder primarily diagnosed in female patients, won inclusion in the revised DSM-III in 1987, in part because of its role in identifying childhood sexual abuse as the primary etiology. Many feminists championed the diagnosis because it dramatized the long-term impacts of early sexual violations. The diagnosis became the site of intense controversy over the therapeutic procedures involved in accessing hidden personalities and exposing the horrifying memories held by these aliens within, separated off from consciousness and emerging during states of mental crisis. For clinicians trained in diagnosing MPD, everything from eating disorders and depressive states, to histrionic and psychotic reactions could signal a communication from the traumatic past via a hidden personality. The recovered memory movement and the expansion of multiple personality disorder treatment programs in the 1990s generated a backlash—institutional efforts to reign in what many viewed as public hysteria over child sexual abuse (Loftus & Ketcham, 1996). DSM-IV sub-committees responded to the crisis with new codes for disentangling valid psychiatric syndromes from their various look-alike simulacra. In DSM-IV, research on PTSD's diagnostic affinity with MPD led to a tightening of criteria, particularly with respect to dissociation—the clinical concept that had been central to explaining the two conditions. The compromise—a standard feature of DSM negotiations—was to create a sub-type: PTSD "with dissociative symptoms." As adjunct to these reform efforts, Spitzer and colleagues (2007) proposed introducing the term "Post-traumatic Stress Injury" to bring the condition more into alignment with the original focus on combat veterans. Qualifiers abounded in the long list of revised criteria and sub-criteria. If trauma diagnoses had reached a fever pitch of hysteria during the previous era, the DSM-5 heralded the reign of the obsessives. Many hairs were split in efforts to refine the PTSD category.

The crusading aspects of the recovered memory movement and the therapeutic authority accompanying excavation of trauma memories produced considerable blindness to the generativity of the human mind (Haaken, 1998). The discovery that recollections reflect the context of their retrieval and that the mind itself is a very creative place ended the epidemic of multiple personality disorder cases with their dramatic choreographies and recovered memories of horrific early abuse. PTSD was the survivor of the memory wars—one that had escaped suspicions of group hysteria. Debates in the literature over veterans who invent military histories, those who imagine battles never fought, raise similar questions about the boundary between fact and fiction, memory and imagination, in the construction of the past (Echterhoff & Hirst, 2009; Frueh, Hamner, Cahill, Gold, & Hamlin, 2000; McNally, 2003). Although noted as a phenomenon associated with veterans' PTSD claims (with widely varying estimates of its frequency), the phenomenon of false memories of veterans has not generated the same scrutiny as did women's reports of child sexual abuse in the 1990s.

Although MPD survived in DSM-5 (American Psychiatric Association, 2013) under the rubric of dissociative identity disorder (DID), the criteria for diagnosis were revised to include recognition of cultural factors: Criterion D requires that the disturbance is not a normal part of a broadly accepted cultural or religious practice. But how broadly accepted must a practice be and who decides on its normalcy? The distinction between a private and a shared delusional system does carry some validity in the diagnosis of psychoses. The clinical difference between the raving paranoid and the ranting preacher occupying the same street corners may very well center on which one can summon an audience of believers. And this difference holds some validity in that the ability to navigate within a shared social reality is part of what constitutes normalcy. But obscured in this DSM caveat on culture is the role of mental health culture itself in the epidemic of MPD cases in the late 20th century (Haaken, 1998).

## Pathologies of Protectors

Although conservative groups enlist the PTSD diagnosis to secure legitimacy for a cause, for example, the specious "post-abortion trauma syndrome" (Dadlez & Andrews, 2010), PTSD has primarily been the psychiatric offspring of progressive movements. The case for protecting the diagnosis is based on accepting the rules imposed by the DSM Committee, however, which are based on individual symptomatology. DSM researcher Robert McNally (2009) describes the expansion of the disorder under DSM-IV and the problem of "conceptual bracket creep." This bracket creep signifies PTSD's perpetual slide into sociology as well—an area psychiatry enters uneasily and unprepared. The rash of PTSD claims related to seeing the collapse of the Trade Towers on 9/11 is cited as an illustration of this creep—one that became a rushing tide in response to the surge of PTSD diagnoses based on watching television reports. The DSM-5 committee specified that the experience must be "first-hand, repeated, or extreme exposure to aversive details of the traumatic event (not through media, pictures, television or movies unless work-related)" (American Psychiatric Association, 2013, p. 217).

Among the powerful social forces driving revisions of PTSD in the 1980s were campaigns against child abuse and woman battering. As these campaigns converged to produce new legislation on domestic violence, advocates advanced findings that children may suffer PTSD symptoms after witnessing domestic violence, along with their mothers who are most commonly the direct victim. The DSM-III definition adopted in 1980 defined a traumatic stressor (Criterion A) as "an event that is outside the range of normal human experience and that would be markedly distressing to almost anyone." DSM-IV tightened the definition of a traumatic stressor to a life-threatening event but loosened criteria for how directly the person is required to have experienced the event. Terms such as "confronted," "witnessed," and "experienced" were used in describing the position of victims to events.

Although PTSD had from the beginning possessed a notable protean quality, a clinical flexibility that lent itself to a wide range of symptom profiles, the diagnosis also required exclusionary rules—clinical indicators that separated the condition from related disorders. Not every trauma could meet Criterion A. Yet this criterial linchpin of the diagnosis reflected the power of specific campaigns and lobbying efforts on the DSM committees. The DSM-IV language that incorporated witnessing violence was in response to new legislation in the United States that included witnessing domestic violence as a condition for reporting child abuse. By the 1990s, most states had expanded reporting laws to include these suspected cases. Parents, even the victims of domestic assaults, could be subject to criminal charges if they allowed their children to remain in situations where they were exposed to violence. This legislation produced confrontations between child advocacy and women's advocacy organizations in expanding the reach of the law into areas where feminists had fought for clear boundaries between male perpetrators and female victims. When mothers failed to intervene in protecting their children from either direct or indirect violence, they could lose custody of those children (Haaken, 2010).

The expansion of child protection laws and parental behaviors considered traumatogenic was an important social advance. Rather than suffering in silence, children subjected to familial violence—including seeing their mothers brutalized by the men in the household—could make claims on the state for protection. Yet modes of remedy and reparation lagged far behind interventions, particularly for poor and minority families. The literature on rates of PTSD among foster children serves as one prime example. Children taken from violent homes often fare no better when under the care of the state. Research consistently reports high rates of PTSD among foster youth, as a result of both their family histories and the conditions of foster care, with some studies reporting rates over four times that of combat veterans (Pecora, White, Jackson, & Wiggins, 2009). Yet the trauma tales of these youth—tales that include the failures of child protection agencies, schools, foster parents, and other caregivers—tend to exceed the capacities of available listeners. Trauma stories represent a social demand—a claim on society for protection or support. But the stories require receptive listeners. The accounts of youth traumatized by the failures of the state periodically capture media attention, only to fade from sight. Further, the PTSD narrative doesn't readily map onto the complicated picture and remote bureaucracies that determine the child's fate.

## Group Transference and Countertransference

In an interview with psychiatrist Robert Jay Lifton, literary theorist Cathy Caruth (2014) notes their mutual attentiveness to the role of symbolization in trauma reactions. Psychic trauma results from situations that exceed available mental resources for representing events and for integrating them into consciousness. The posttraumatic experience of emotional numbing signals the gap between the event and mental representational resources, an "impairment in the symbolization process itself" (p. 9). From this perspective, empathic listening is a creative act. The therapist assists the traumatized person in constructing coherence and meaning from what is initially experienced as a deathly void. "And as one forms imagery, one is forming a narrative about their story," Caruth explains. "It's all forming itself or being reconstructed, recreated in the symbolizing process of the therapist" (p. 17). My interest here is in how social dynamics structure this symbolizing process.

In this section, I describe some of those dynamics as they operate on the institutional level for military clinicians and stress control teams. In the Army's combat readiness training, leaders are attuned to their roles in helping soldiers construct a story about warfare that stays mission-focused. The leader of an all-day training session, filmed as part of my documentary field work, described how he found his own motivational story in the movies. For this instructor, *Rocky* spoke most directly to pitfalls in the negative thinking that can undermine psychological resilience. "Rocky had a ton of thinking traps, right? He was blaming everybody and everything except for himself." Identifying himself with Rocky's dad in the movie, he offers that "Rocky's dad was telling his son to quit being a baby, life is hard" (M. R. T. Anderson, personal communication, March 15, 2011).

Mental health providers in Afghanistan also note that life in war zones is hard, but they also know the limits of the power of positive thinking. Their stories more often referenced *Catch 22* and *MASH*, works about the absurd irrationalities of military culture. One psychiatrist with the 113th Medical Detachment in Afghanistan shared with me an anecdote about a soldier caught in a Catch-22:

> I had a soldier who had been in three different ambushes in a week. I asked that he be taken off the line for a week. The commander said "No, we need him." The soldier then took a cinder block and broke his foot. And then the commander was calling me saying "What should I do?" I said, "Your decision, your call. It looks like its five years in prison for a self-inflicted wound to get out of duty or ten years in a combat zone."
>
> (personal communication, July 2, 2011)

But the psychiatrist found himself in this same Catch-22. He had made a psychiatric recommendation that was rejected by the commander. But in this new situation, the self-inflicted injury required a more elaborate psychological explanation to protect the soldier from disciplinary action. Line-of-duty injuries are routinely investigated in the military because they are very common and red flags for commanders worried about evacuation rates. Psychiatrists have played leading roles since World War I in assessing soldiers under suspicion for producing symptoms in order to escape military service.

In my field interviews, clinicians explained why service members were not assigned a psychiatric diagnosis while in theater. One of the rationales dates back to World War I and what is described as the "evacuation syndrome." The syndrome is a group reaction, thought to be a variant of war neurosis, where soldiers develop symptoms as they see one of the members of their unit evacuated for psychiatric treatment. The sight of a comrade delivered from danger destabilizes the tenuous suppression and/or repression of the conscious wish to escape. During World War I, doctors reported patterns of shell-shock symptoms that were endemic to particular units, with some physicians concluding that patients either consciously or unconsciously learned to mimic the characteristic palsied movements of other soldiers. Otto Binswanger, a leading psychiatrist in the literature on war neuroses during World War I, introduced group identifications into his classification system. He distinguished between the "acute hystericization" of soldiers in wake of battlefield experiences and "front hysteria" or "field-hospital hysteria" caused by social psychological factors, including empathy or identification with other injured soldiers and mimicry (Binswanger, 1922). Yet, this distinction generated little interest in the social psychology of war neuroses beyond separating the "true cases" from the simulated displays that were subject to military discipline.

This same controversy over "contagion" effects arose with scrutiny of the Gulf War syndrome in the early 1990s. Family members began to exhibit some of the same physical and emotional symptoms as those of returning veterans. While exposure to toxins was at the center of explanations advanced by veterans' groups, the appointed investigative panels concluded that there was no single Gulf War syndrome and that many of the symptoms could be attributed to PTSD (Kang & Bullman, 1996). Veterans' groups vehemently rejected government research reports, incensed that their infirmities were interpreted as psychological rather than physiological.

The Gulf War syndrome aligned with the pre-PTSD syndromes, such as concentration camp syndrome and Vietnam syndrome, in its affiliation with an historical event and its acknowledged clinical ambiguity. The controversy signaled a departure, however, from the late 20th-century trajectory of PTSD as a "good diagnosis," a condition that shed the stigma attached to other mental disorders. Most veterans' groups rejected this explanation for their troubles. For them, the diagnosis was a government cover-up that denied what they insisted to be biological and chemical causes of their symptoms. The military investigative panel was careful in describing the conditions of Gulf veterans as stress reactions and in normalizing their responses. Since most of the veterans were spared direct combat, the panel cited evidence of how anticipatory anxiety—occupying the garrison position in war zones—can be as traumatic as direct exposure to combat. PTSD had been embraced by Vietnam veterans as an acknowledgment of their delayed reactions to the trauma of war. But in the case of the Gulf War, veterans refused the government-issued term for their symptoms—a fight that continues close to two decades later (Kime, 2016).

We can see how group dynamics and societal responses to the war contributed to the clinical picture. As the border between Iraq and Kuwait was pounded from the air, the US-led coalition declared victory after just 100 hours of ground war. Described as the first "video game war," in reference to the satellite images circulating non-stop on television, the Gulf War was itself dissociated from public consciousness. The surreal aspects of the military assault extended into the post-war media displays of victory and the absence of any memorializing or acknowledgment of the large-scale slaughter. As historian

Marita Sturken (1997) explains, the Persian Gulf War "is a war about which Americans, even during the war itself, were perceived to have a collective amnesia" (p. 122). She goes on to explain how the syndromes of this war must be understood in the context of "the sanitized public story of the war." The military intervention was produced for the screen as a display of military power before a global audience—a performance intended to bring an end to the Vietnam syndrome and its extension into the helplessness associated with the Iranian hostage crisis. Indeed, George H. W. Bush declared triumphantly at the close of the Gulf War that "the Vietnam Syndrome is over!" One of the lessons—an aspect of the "syndrome"—centered on controlling the way the story of war gets told. Media were embedded with military units and provided no observational distance from the war. Two iconic images took hold for their signifying power—the bombs over the night sky of Baghdad and the point of view of the "smart-bomb" hitting its target. Unlike the photos that came out of the Vietnam War, with their human scale anguish, the Persian Gulf War was eerily unpeopled (Sturken, 1997).

Since the PTSD diagnosis carries such a heavy load of political history, the adjudication of claims around its use is inevitably fraught. But we may recognize how Gulf War veterans who suffered neurological conditions that left them emaciated could acquire signifying power as representative of the unrecognized impacts of that conflict. There may indeed by interactive effects that produce a disorder, from exposure to toxins, personal vulnerabilities, and a host of other factors. The research panel identified a much larger group of psychosomatic veterans—those with physical complaints but no clear medical diagnosis. But psychiatric diagnoses, including PTSD, offer no way of honorably accounting for symptoms based on identifications with impaired comrades. As Binswanger noted during World War I, bonds of sympathy and identification can be expressed through shared symptoms. If PTSD is really about disturbances in the memory of an event—reactions dislocated from their temporal frame—we might recognize how these same dynamics operate on a collective level. As the symptom bearers of that conflict, veterans themselves carry a culturally unmetabolized load of loss, grief, and rage.

## The Rape Survivor Movement

Second-wave feminists played important roles in the choreography of trauma conditions that led to the DSM-III adoption of PTSD. Rape survivors shared with veterans a sense of outrage over dismissal of their grievances, including psychiatrists summoned to evaluate their claims. Yet a striking difference between the stories of rape survivors and those of veterans centers on the allowance granted service members for the expression of ambivalence. John King's story told in Chapter 1 is rife with the love/hate attachment to the military—and acknowledgment that "when you do good, commanders notice." Rape stories center on shame and self-doubt. Support groups were a vital part of

Second-wave feminist efforts to cast off these debilitating states, including being cast as "damaged goods." Identification with the aggressor figured prominently in the Abraham and Isaac narrative of the soldiers' trauma. But accounts of rape survivors allowed for little of this psychological complexity, in part because the woman's conflicts had been so routinely used historically to discredit her testimony (Haaken, 2010, 2017).

There were feminists in the rape survivor movement who took up the cultural choreography of rape, however, and insisted on a more complex story. In her discussion of Second-wave sexual politics, Sharon Marcus (2002) argues that "rape is structured like a language" (p. 390), and so is the narrative that structures its aftermath. "The horror of rape," Marcus argues, "is not that it steals something from us but it makes us into things to be taken" (p. 399). Rather than conceiving of female sexuality as a "fixed spatial unit," she continues, "think of it in terms of time and change." Marcus cautions against enlisting the term *invasion* as a metaphor for rape because it reproduces this dichotomy between inner (feminine) and outer (masculine) spaces. She cites feminist researchers who argue that many rape survivors do not conceptualize it as an invasion but rather as the "extraction of a service" (p. 399)—as making the woman do something for him. She points out how little talk there is of the vulnerability of the erect penis—how women have been able to grab it and stop the man in his act of violence.

Another feminist challenge taken up by Second-wave feminism centered on the rape drama as one where the woman was overwhelmed by the sheer power of her assailant. The best strategy, girls and women were instructed, was to remain still and passive. In published findings in the 1980s, Pauline Bart and Patricia O'Brien (1985) challenge the conventional wisdom that fighting back makes women more vulnerable to injury. They conclude that women who push, shove, or hit their assailant are more apt to disrupt rape. They also took on the traditional focus on female verbal skills, of talking men out of it—a script closely aligned with the feminine position of taming the beast, domesticating her man.

In the early 1990s, Kimberle Crenshaw (1991, 1992) introduced the concept of intersectionality to critique Eurocentric feminist models that over-universalize and over-simplify links between gender and sexual violence. She emphasizes the dynamic interplay of systems of oppression in shaping women's experiences of violence—and that any system of domination produces forms of violence. While white women may suffer severe penalties for violating moral and sexual codes, black women have never been protected by the powerful patriarchs (Collins, 2000; hooks, 1982). But the critique of black feminists extends beyond this differential treatment—their more fundamental lack of protection—to the complicity of white women in racist storytelling. White women's outrage over rape, their conviction that this was the worst of crimes against humanity, may easily overlook the racist history of sexual allegations. When Susan Brownmiller's (1975/2005) groundbreaking book on

rape was taken up by feminists in the 1970s, with rape emerging as the prototype of women's oppression generally, some feminists, such as bell hooks,
criticized her ahistorical understanding of sexual violence and her failure to
address the racist history behind allegations of rape.

Bringing the wider social context into the picture helps in unpacking the
frequently repeated finding that 25 percent of college women have experienced
either rape or attempted rape. First, this finding collapses important distinctions
along a continuum from rape to sexual interactions that may include pressure,
insensitivity, and poor communication. Collapsing attempted and completed
acts loses sight of resistance to rape and the role of female solidarity in fighting back.

The bystander intervention programs that have gained currency have
expanded the lens of sexual assault, going beyond the victim/perpetrator
dyad and bringing into focus group contexts of sexual violence (McMahon
et al., 2015). Many of these campaigns—including online videos and signing
pledges—enlarge the moral field of responsibility. The "It's on us" campaign
is one such example: "It's on us to look out for each other, to not look the
other way, to not blame the victims. It's on us—all of us—to stop sexual
assault." In moving beyond victim/perpetrator interactions, students are asked
to make a pledge not to remain a passive bystander (Banyard, Moynihan, &
Plante, 2007).

From a psychoanalytic feminist perspective, bystander interventions allow
for a more complex group psychology of violence than the stereotypical script
of (and splitting between) the all-good victim and all-bad perpetrator positions that often accompany abuse allegations (Gentile, 2015). Bystander programs provide a context for identification with both perpetrator and victim and
introduce the importance of what psychoanalysis calls the "third term"—the
observer position that permits perspective-taking and more complex forms of
identification and moral responsibility (see Benjamin, 2018). With the widespread endorsement of the bystander model, it's easy to overlook, however, the
class and race politics of the classic studies that gave this term such currency.

In one of the classic bystander studies of the late 1960s, the Kitty Genovese
study, researchers interviewed neighbors in a New York City tenement building who had observed a woman being killed in the street below, inquiring as to
why they had failed to intervene or call the police. In telling their stories, most
observers of the violence explained that they had assumed that someone else
would intervene. The social psychological phenomenon that emerged from this
study was termed *diffusion of responsibility*. After subsequent investigation of
the conditions under which people intervene, researchers concluded that the
fewer the observers, the more likely the victim will receive aid from bystanders
(Latané & Darley, 1970).

In her analysis of the construction of the Kitty Genovese story as a social
psychological phenomenon, Carrie Rentschler (2011) reviews many of the
inaccuracies in the original reporting that continue to be included in social

psychology textbooks. The report of 38 people passively watching as a woman is raped and murdered outside of her apartment has achieved the status of a collective memory, inscribed with the fantasies and fears of the era. The person of Kitty Genovese herself—as a lesbian Italian woman who confronted a mentally ill stranger on her way home from work—has been virtually erased by the centrality of the passive observer story. Her murder became a story of urban anomie and crime fear cast against an emergent racialized threat construction and, by the late 1960s, federally deployed discourses that defined criminality as "Black" and "of the street." Sitting on the cusp of the 1968 declaration of a US war on crime, the murder of Kitty Genovese offered a narrative of crime where the victim and the scene of the crime functioned as a backdrop, a facial screen and mask against which another collectivized face, that of the 38 witnesses, would be projected. The fact that there were six or seven rather than 38 observers to the crime, and that many neighbors had tried to call the police but gave up because the police were unresponsive to their calls, complicates this morality tale (Griggs & Whitehead, 2015).

## The Penitentiary and Penitence

Whether a prisoner at the Oregon State Penitentiary or a patient at the Oregon State Hospital next door, incarcerated persons learn rhetorical conventions for telling trauma stories and for gauging what audiences are receptive to hearing. PTSD centers on a story where the victim of an event need not feel implicated in its occurrence nor in the symptoms that result. But for prisoners, the PTSD story finds a cold reception. The emphasis on crime victims is a centerpiece of Restorative Justice classes at OSP, as well as in other programs focused on alternatives to law-and-order approaches to crime. The programs reject the punitive premises of the criminal justice system and envision ways of bringing rule-violators back into a human community rather than shunning them or casting them as inherently evil. Restorative Justice also emphasizes the humanity of perpetrators and their capacity for change. One of the members of the Lifers Club at OSP, a group that I met with over a period of a year, describes in a newsletter sent to community supporters the importance of coming to terms with the impact of his own act of killing:

> We often can't visualize what the extreme actions have done to affect the families that we essentially destroy. . . . In any case of a traumatic incident, the imagery of our violent actions play out in a never-ending cycle that plays over and over in our minds like a terminal illness.
> (OSP Lifers Club, December Newsletter, 2017)

The club took seriously the decision of when and to whom to tell the stories of their crimes, including in sessions with victims who agree to participate in dialogues with former perpetrators.

The truth of a story and its believability often depend on the audience. For those with indeterminate sentences, presenting to the parole board requires skills in demonstrating what parole boards term "insight"—taking responsibility for your crime. But insight in this context excludes references to the prisoners' own traumatic past. While the PTSD patient is relieved of responsibility for harms suffered, the prisoner is tasked with taking full individual responsibility for crimes. Any reference to the role of others in the crime, to societal forces, or to abuses or poverty suffered in childhood, signals to parole boards that the inmate lacks insight. Lilliana Paratore (2016) describes what she terms the "rhetoric of remorse" and how demands for demonstration of "insight" are used to justify extending prison terms by parole boards. The narrowly choreographed and institutionally authorized scripts over-ride the personal histories of inmates, including histories of personal trauma. Paratore adds that this "rhetoric of remorse" reflects the "tension between dominant notions of the inmate as intrinsically criminal and as having the potential to be rehabilitated and reformed" (p. 98). Advocates of those seeking parole have begun to challenge the use of clinicians hired by the Board of Parole Hearings and the arbitrary nature of their assessments of psychopathy (Tangney, Stuewig, & Hafez, 2011). The California Innocence Project describes the Catch-22 of this demand, and particularly for prisoners wrongly convicted: "they cannot accept responsibility for a crime they did not commit, but they will never be granted parole if they do not" (California Innocence Project, 2019)

Psychoanalysis teaches that even valuable ideas can be used defensively. Focusing on internal dynamics can be a means of avoiding or disavowing external factors and vice versa. The PTSD diagnosis orients attention to external causes of symptoms, although within a narrowly drawn field of determinants. Psychoanalysis attends to internal dynamics—to areas of conflict and how they are shaped by formative relationships and experiences. Because women have a longer history as patients than do men and have been more intimately subjected to psychiatric scrutiny, the externalizing bias of the PTSD diagnosis can feel liberating. The diagnosis offers a form of redemption by locating the source of a problem onto an external powerful actor. For the oppressed, turning from a debilitating internal state of shame and guilt and pointing an accusatory finger at the enemy can feel therapeutic. And for veterans escaping the psychological yoke of the military, it can feel similarly freeing to proclaim, "I'm not a loser, it was the war that fucked me up." The question here centers on the costs of such defenses over time and which aspects of experience are perpetually cast to the margins of consciousness in the process.

## Group Dynamics and War Stories

A group of veterans we filmed one summer evening in 2011, shortly before our crew left for Afghanistan, confronted me with a question as we were setting up for the shoot. Most were Vietnam War veterans, and they agreed to be part of the *Mind Zone* documentary on the word of John King, a lead subject in the film. The veterans gathered weekly at a pub in Gresham, a working-class town east of Portland on the highway leading up to Mount Hood. The vets—nine or ten men and one woman (a former Marine Corps nurse)—met regularly over beers as a kind of informal support group. John held deep respect for these older veterans and the feeling was clearly mutual. But I was an outsider, and the question arose of how this footage of their discussions would be used. "What were you doing during the Vietnam War?" one surly veteran wearing a Marine Corps baseball cap demanded. "Were you one of those protestors spitting on veterans?" he added with a confrontational stare. He had profiled me on the spot. I responded with the simplest version of the truth that came to mind: "Yes, I was involved in protesting the Vietnam War, but no, I did not believe in behaving disrespectfully to returning solders." This response seemed to satisfy, although I wondered about the image of the spitting pro-testors. The story had acquired the status of folk legend among veterans. In talking with this group, it also became clear that many were themselves spitting-mad. The focus of their anger shifted fluidly over the course of the evening from protesters, Vietnam, the military brass, and the VA bureaucracy to the broader society. The various contemporary war syndromes, from the post-Vietnam syndrome and Gulf War syndrome to PTSD, seem to share this diffuse and labile anger, a weapon in search of its target, which sometimes becomes the veteran himself.

In the discussion at the pub, the emotional tenor of the conversation softened over the course of the evening, perhaps because of the beers or feeling more at ease with the film crew, or because many of these veterans are now grand-parents. The conversation moved from their various war experiences to what the American culture teaches young people about killing. One of the veterans took up key points from *On Killing*, the book by psychologist and Major Dave Grossman (2009). This Vietnam-era veteran emphasized that he was not a peacenik, but he agreed with Grossman's thesis that military training centers on overcoming soldiers' inhibitions against the use of lethal violence.

The shift from pro-war to anti-war sentiments among service members was to be a recurring motif throughout the documentary project—a sentiment tan-gled up in ambivalence about the military itself. While distinctions between various wars shape generational identities, veterans of different eras express the conviction that war changes a person. It leaves an irreducible remain-der of distress that is hard to integrate into other aspects of one's life and mind, whether the veteran meets criteria for a stress condition or not. As one infantryman told me, "The most antiwar people you're gonna find are in the infantry." Indeed, it seems to be quite common for service members to love the military and hate its wars. And with an all-volunteer army, the new caring ethos of the US military has been a driving force in recruiting and maintain-ing the fighting force—seductive appeals to young men and women hungry for recognition.

As now Retired Colonel David Rabb, Commander of the 113th Combat Stress Control unit, often reminded me, "there is a lot of love in the military." The old image of the barking drill sergeant is now outdated, he added, a stereotype that he claims lives on primarily in the movies. And his own ideal as a social worker and reservist embodies this new military ethos of care and love. He talks about growing up as a black kid in South Side Chicago, deeply attached to his mother and a self-described "mama's boy." The world outside of this protective maternal fold was harsh. Joining the Marines armed him for a world that was armed against him. He recalls being taken to jail and booked at the age of 8. The police had gotten a call about vandalism in his neighborhood and picked him up as a random black kid playing in the area. Later joining the Army reserves, Colonel Rabb got a lot from the military: college and graduate training as a social worker, recognition and respect, and a sense of personal power tempered by religious conviction and the Soldier's Creed.

After retiring from the Army, Rabb brutally encountered the limits of that love and the illusions of its protective reach. After suffering a stroke and being hospitalized for months, Rabb learned that his wife had been questioned by an Army investigator about whether Rabb may have done something during his post-deployment assignments to cause his own stroke. He was still on active duty as a reservist at the Palo Alto VA's Polytrauma Center. Although the Army insisted that line-of-duty investigations are routine to determine whether a medical incident or injury was the result of negligence or bad judgment on the part of the soldier, Rabb was emotionally shattered when he learned of this inquiry. After decades of exemplary service and of extending his tour to cover a shortage of mental health staff, Rabb felt like a discarded asset. He petitioned to have moral injury added to his medical record—a term that conveyed the depth of his sense of betrayal. The panel of commanders at Joint Base Lewis–McChord where he presented his case insisted that the inquiry was routine, although clearly done in a highly insensitive manner. Rabb countered that the inquiry was systematic of a deeper problem in the Army. He also presented a case that this kind of insensitive treatment was consistent with a larger pattern of racism in the Army's command structure (D. Rabb, personal communications, November 8 and 24, 2019).

As a high-ranking officer, Rabb was unique in coming forward to tell this story in a way that exposed his feelings of betrayal and abandonment. A Soldier and former Marine, Rabb understood toughness. But his military identity was more oriented toward caring than killing. Soldiers had a clear duty to watch out for one another, and this buddyship operated as the most basic psychological principle of military life. But the creed also lionized stoicism: Never giving up, never quitting, and never turning back on the mission—values that led him to continue to fill in for the Army even after he had completed his deployment and returned to his civilian job. In talking with Rabb on several occasions about this agonizing time, I questioned whether moral injury was the best term for what happened to him. Although he had the right to call it whatever he chose,

I asked him whether the concept of moral injury left something important behind in that experience—something perhaps that he had kept out of mind during service but was now attempting to integrate into his ideal of the military as a nurturing institution. For Rabb, moral injury, or "wound to the soul," remained the best way of describing the cause of his psychiatric breakdown that followed—his hospitalization for suicidal ideation and acute depression—because it kept the focus on harms inflicted by the military. For Rabb, moral injury was less of a metaphor than a concrete physical reality. Yet whatever the term, he had suffered a loss of faith in an institution that had anchored his very sense of being. But we agreed that the language of wounds and injury was required for the military to actually see the violations he suffered.

The burgeoning field of moral injury grew from an effort to empirically assess the claims of military critics that the effects of warfare are deep and lasting. The field has produced an array of instruments to measure this construct and to incorporate these measures into post-war assessments and debates over whether the Moral Injury Events Scale (MIES) is a two- or three-factor scale (Nash & Litz, 2013). The appeal of this construct—most notably in how it has been assimilated into Department of Defense manuals and their lists of psychological risks in military service—registers its utility as an institutional symptom. The concept both targets a source of anxiety for the military and military clinicians and creates the illusion of a means of bringing it under control.

While the PTSD symptom list includes trouble with the law, the emotional states associated with this trouble tend to be downplayed (Brown, 2008). The Vietnam syndrome, precursor to PTSD, was a condition characterized by alienation and anger (Shay, 1994). As David Cortright (1975) notes in his history of GI resistance during the Vietnam War, anger was pervasive among service members and a unifying emotion in resistance to the war. As the PTSD movement claimed new ground in addressing the long-term effects of war, individual symptoms and treatment strategies took center stage. The specific struggles of veterans—and the forms of collective identity and camaraderie created through shared experiences—were repressed in the totalizing and universalizing logic of PTSD. Even emotional symptoms associated with the disorder shifted, with helplessness and fear dominating the clinical picture rather than anger. The moral injury literature has attempted to capture some of the emotional remainder left behind by DSM constraints on PTSD even as it depends on the diagnosis itself for status as the "deeper" companion condition ("The Shay Moral Injury Center," n.d.).

The early PTSD stories did allow for ambivalence about the military and about being part of the war machine. A baseline principle of military culture centers on preparedness for killing. The outrage of soldiers often involves being drawn into senseless killing—or killing for an unworthy cause. As Mohammad Ali stated it in refusing in 1967 to fight during the Vietnam War: "No, I am not going ten thousand miles from home to help murder and burn another poor nation simply to continue the domination of white slave masters of the darker people the world over." But as the war continued and a GI move-ment of resisters grew, atrocities became a key signifier of the dark night of the soldier's soul. The Winter Soldier Investigation—one of the early anti-war media interventions—brought onto the public stage accounts of soldiers engaged in horrific brutality, extending the scandal over the My Lai massacre to the broader landscape of the war. Chaim Shatan (1989) a psychiatrist with the Vietnam Veterans Working Group, draws on Freud's theory of grief and mourning in his vivid, lyrical accounts of the post-Vietnam syndrome: "Their sorrow is unspent, the grief of their wounds is untold, their guilt unexpiated" (p. 136). While veterans had gathered since the Revolutionary War to swap buddy stories and complain about commanders, Vietnam vets expressed a col-lective outrage that carried a long post-war echo.

## Psychoanalysis and Intergenerational Trauma

As clinicians confront the limits of the PTSD paradigm and its diagnostic con-straints, the concept of intergenerational trauma holds elements of the early movement's focus on the long-term effects of warfare. In the anti-war move-ment, the diagnosis emerged as a call to remember and a form of resistance to collective forms of forgetting. The emphasis on delayed symptoms—the notion that the mental effects of warfare could appear years or decades after the close of a conflict—represented more of a rhetorical strategy than a medical claim. As psychiatrist and trauma theorist Judith Herman (2017) describes the early political project, the aim was to counter the culture of silence and denial surrounding victim claims. Perpetrators invoke repressive appeals to "move on" after war, rape, or atrocities in the interest of keeping the peace. "The incidents should never be discussed and preferably they should be forgotten altogether," Herman explains in characterizing this code of silence. But as the diagnosis secured a position in the DSM and weathered various challenges to its reliability and validity, the metaphors became increasingly concrete. Poetics gave way to protocols.

The Holocaust occupies a revered place in trauma theory as an event that defies clinical categorization and serves as a lighthouse projecting a range of signals. Fred Alford (2009) takes up the famous proclamation by Theodor Adorno (1967) that "there can be no poetry after Auschwitz" to point out that there can be no silence after Auschwitz, either. The representational crisis that generations of trauma theorists have confronted centers on the moral demand to "bear witness" to trauma, on the one hand, and to avoid the linguistic vio-lence of formulaic witnessing, on the other. In writing about the ethical chal-lenges in working with the stories of Holocaust survivors, Alford cautions against the impulse to create narrative coherence or closure out of survivors' accounts (Alford, 2009).

Critics have pointed out the bias in psychiatry toward a one-person psychology and how this bias blinds practitioners to social and interactive dimensions of diagnostic processes (Gone, 2014). Some clinical traditions have conceptualized psychopathology as an interactive dynamic within a social field rather than as a condition of individual psyches. R.D. Laing. (1967), a leading theorist of the anti-psychiatry movement, approached psychopathology within a nexus of social relations rather than as a disturbance of individual psyches. Laing contributed to the field of family systems theory, for example, in recognizing that one person in a family could serve as the "identified patient" or "symptom-bearer" for others (Crossley, 1998). The field of family systems therapy, for example, grew out of recognition that one person in a family could serve as the "identified patient" or "symptom-bearer" for others, including in the enactment of traumatic experiences. Parents may unconsciously set up a child to enact a script, attempting to bring the child (and a deviant part of themselves) under control while vicariously identifying with the tabooed behavior. The dutiful and submissive mother may unconsciously reinforce a wild daughter, for example, through the intergenerational transmission of unconscious defiance. Or that same dutiful mother may produce a feminist daughter, talking back when the mother is inclined to bite her tongue. Therapists working in war zones also describe how a soldier may act out the problems of the unit—a dynamic taken up in Chapter 1.

As an intergenerational dynamic, traumatic reactions can take the form of each generation taking up the lost battles of elders or fleeing this same site of conflict in a reaction formation—a defense that involves over-compensating by taking on behaviors that hold a countervailing impulse in check. Psycho-analysts have written, for example, about the bravado and hyper-masculinity that became normative in post-war Israel in reaction to accounts of their elders being led to their slaughter. In her discussion of gender dynamics associated with Zionism, legal scholar Karin Carmin Yefet (2016) explains how "the New Jew was to become 'a superhuman,' one socially engineered to respond to the inferior image of the old Jew by engaging in hyper-masculine perfor-mances that would take the Zionism's New Jew from 'zero to a hero'" (p. 58). Therapists approaching intergenerational trauma through the lens of family dynamics describe a familial division of emotional labor where overwhelm-ing experiences, events that go beyond what is representable, for example, are unconsciously broken into fragmented parts and carried by individual family members in the psychiatric or physical symptoms in offspring.

In the course of reviewing a film by psychoanalytic therapist Molly Castel-loe (2019) titled *Vamik's Room*, I revisited the work of Vamik Volkan, undoubt-edly the most recognized psychoanalyst working globally in conflict zones (Haaken, 2018). Rather than invoking parental pathology as the sites for the intergenerational transmission of trauma, Volkan focuses on large group iden-tity. In the film, Volkan suggests that large group identity is like "a second skin. It's part of our nature. You are born into it—like mother's milk. . . . If someone scratches your skin, your core is humiliated, you need to protect it."

Volkan's work centers on how real and imagined trauma bind groups in conflict zones around the world. His concept of *chosen trauma* explains how communities that have suffered war and displacements do enlist representations of historical events to justify acts of aggression. Volkan observes how nationalism depends on mobilizing a traumatic event in history at the level of large group identity (Volkan, 1998). These are appeals to reclaim that which has been lost, accompanied by aggrieved entitlement. The charismatic appeal of nationalist leaders depends on their ability to revisit and revive ancient losses—a defeat in battle or lost territory—and to respond as though this injury to the large group constitutes a current and ever-present threat (Volkan, 2001). Volkan enlists the concept of *time collapse* to describe this near delusional sense of immediacy (Volkan, 1999).

The formulations of Volkan suggest a collective syndrome analogous to post-traumatic stress disorder. In the cases he presents, authoritarian leaders revive emotionally charged images in the nation's past that have acquired socially symbolic meaning, for example, a statue or a painting of a battle fought centuries prior. The disturbing elements of the nation's history are projected onto an outsider group—which may be people living inside the borders of this same country. The leader attributes the disturbing parts of the national history onto this outsider group—a defense that protects the leader and the majority group from internal conflict and produces a state of shared idealization. The "bad" parts of the in-group are displaced onto the outsider group—a defense that produces an illusory field of protection. The dynamic described by Volkan operates much like the image of the scapegoat in the book of Leviticus:

> He is to lay both hands on the head of the live goat and confess over it all the wickedness and rebellion of the Israelites—all their sins—and put them on the goat's head. He shall send the goat away into the wilderness in the care of someone appointed for the task. The goat will carry on itself all their sins to a remote place; and the man shall release it in the wilderness.
>
> (Leviticus 16:21, New International Version)

Volkan explains how collective conflicts are dynamic and in flux, just as are individual psyches. Borders between groups and countries are similarly in states of flux. This dynamic approach to international conflict opens possibilities for new resolutions. Volkan emphasizes that "ethno-hatreds" are not inscribed in group identities in a fixed way. Ancient enmities are not simply stored unconsciously and then unleashed when the old regime collapses. Rather, memory fragments and affectively charged images are brought together into an emotionally stirring mythology—an ideology of ethno-hatred and fortified borders—that serves the narrow interests of opportunistic leaders. Groups in crisis are often vulnerable to the influence of charismatic leaders and may hold fast to its "chosen trauma"—an event in the past that acquires the status of mythology and operates as rationale for violence.

Yet this question of how old losses are politically revived is far less formulaic than this theory would suggest. In my field research on Lakota psychology and domestic violence on the Pine Ridge Reservation, for example, many of the programs there, such as Sacred Circle, framed the problem of interpersonal violence as a response to intergenerational transmission of cultural trauma (Haaken, 2008b). Activists and counselors routinely referenced the Wounded Knee Massacre of 1889 and the defeat of AIM in the stand-off with the FBI at Wounded Knee in 1973. They argued that the battles of the past continue to be fought in a displaced way through violence within the family. Volkan would most likely see in this Lakota example a progressive use of the traumatic past, an effort to make conscious the potential for re-enacting scenes of traumatic violence. But as we saw with the Standing Rock resistance to the Dakota access pipeline, this same history can open up new calls for political resistance. One of the scenes at Standing Rock that captured the media stage centered on US veterans positioning themselves as shields in protecting Water Protectors from the assaults of the police—scenes that included a moving ceremony where veterans knelt and apologized for the history of violence directed against Indigenous peoples (Levin, 2017).

In *Achilles in Vietnam: Combat Trauma and the Undoing of Character*, Jonathan Shay (1994) enlists classic tragedy in creating narrative coherence out of the tales of anguish, guilt, and betrayal that surfaced in his combat veteran groups. Drawing on Homer's epic poem on the Trojan War, Shay moves between Homer's narrative and the stories of Vietnam veterans shared in therapy groups. He concludes that recovery from combat-related PTSD requires cultural spaces for grieving the losses that accompany warfare, including the loss of the person one was before the war. The failure to "communalize grief can lock a person into chronic rage" (p. 55), Shay observes. Recovery requires developing identifications with former enemies and coming to terms with one's own existential vulnerability.

In much of my academic writing, documentary filmmaking, and activism, I have focused on intrapsychic and social dynamics of guilt (Haaken, 1998, 2002a, 2002b, 2008a, 2008b, 2016, 2017; Haaken & Palmer, 2012; Haaken, Wallin-Ruschman, & Patange, 2012). My line of analysis frequently draws on Kleinian traditions of psychoanalysis—works by Melanie Klein that place awareness of one's capacity for destructiveness at the center of psychology. The capacity for insight requires an ability to reflect on one's roles in the disturbing dramas of life. And it involves attending to the intense ambivalences around attachment, including how former lovers can become the bitterest of enemies. Idealized objects—people or parts of people that represent what is felt to be most precious—are also vulnerable to attack when they disappoint or fail to gratify. Kleinian theory holds useful ideas for thinking about dynamic currents in group life and how groups often depend on enemies and outsider groups in defending against internal anxieties (Haaken, 1998; Alford, 2001; Burack, 2002). But alongside these defensive dynamics, the theory attends to human efforts to make reparation with others. What Kleinians term the *depressive position* describes a process of moral awareness and recognition of harms suffered by others and one's own connection to those harms.

Some of my field work has taken place in refugee camps in West Africa and in settings in the US and Britain where refugees are seeking asylum (Haaken & O'Neill, 2014). In documenting the stories of asylum seekers, Maggie O'Neill and I focused on how migrants and refugees carried images of the world they left behind into the new country. A part of this work addressed reactions in Britain to asylum seekers and how public fantasies, fears, and defenses infuse perceptions of foreigners. Stigmatized groups are often those that perform work upon which others depend, from women's household labor and farm workers to the many undocumented workers who bath, feed, and tend to the bodily needs of other citizens.

The position of asylum seeker is itself often feminized in its association in the public imagination with desperate states of dependency, vulnerability, and need. While men have dominated the ranks of economic migrants historically, several decades of closing the borders for purposes of stopping economic immigration produced a new ideological loading of the claims of asylum seekers, particularly in Britain (O'Neill, 2010). The male asylum seeker is often cast as suspect, as sneaking into the country under the garb of helplessness to suck voraciously on the generous tit of the welfare state. Although women's asylum claims were in the past more apt to be approved than were male claims (Bohmer & Shuman, 2008), the Trump administration dismantled many of the legal protections in the United States granted to women escaping domestic violence and sexual assault in their home countries (Green, 2019).

The asylum seeker's story may be deployed to affirm the beneficence of the state even as the state more aggressively polices borders. Although the 1951 UN Convention Related to the Status of Refugees established the right to seek asylum and criteria for refugee status, that and subsequent provisions in international law also uphold the right of national sovereignty—and the right of nation states to determine whether any particular case meets criteria for asylum. In response to the brutal fortification of borders and the anti-immigrant policies of reactionary regimes in the United States, the UK, and Europe, immigrant rights groups call for more humane asylum policies. But whether hard or soft borders are in place, refugees still confront the demand to produce a compelling story. In the US, the threshold rose in the Trump era as children were separated from their parents at the US/Mexico border and put in cages. But these visceral scenes of cruelty and inhumanity are readily incorporated into a new genre of dramatic stories that reproduce the same dilemmas migrants have long confronted. In bringing the PTSD diagnosis into proceedings, forensic psychiatrists explain to judges why the story may seem contradictory or fragmented. But this strategy accepts as a premise the demand at various disputed border crossings for a dramatic account of suffering to secure passage.

## Conclusions

The PTSD movement grew out of calls among progressive clinicians for a new vision of psychiatry. Animated by the feminist and anti-war campaigns of the

1970s, this vision sought to identify and address the societal origins of many of the symptoms that they were treating. From a psychoanalytic perspective, PTSD procedures for diagnosis foreclose on the accounts that ground suffering in historical and relational contexts as well as in forms of solidarity. Although the PTSD script registers collective forms of suffering, the diagnostic process places societal dynamics on the periphery of the stage. Whatever the promise of a progressive psychiatry and whatever the prospects for a critical psychoanalysis, relying on this expertise to protect people at hostile borders ultimately risks silencing others in the course of helping them.

In working with visual metaphors, I have argued here for a wide-angle lens on suffering. All professions by necessity bring the tools of their trade to their assigned tasks. Those tools inevitably structure elements of the picture of what features become most salient. In taking up PTSD as a tool for clinicians in conflict zones, I have shown its various blind spots and how these holes in the field of vision become more apparent as the reach of the diagnosis extends far beyond its grasp. It's instructive that anthropological psychiatrists have sounded the strongest alarms about the use of this diagnosis and trauma theory more generally in framing the experiences of survivors. However, the wide-angle anthropological or sociological view can mean missing important details in the experiences of survivors.

## References

Adorno, T. W. (1967). *Prisms* (S. W. Nicholsen & S. Weber, Trans.). Cambridge, MA: The MIT Press.

Alford, C. F. (2001). *Melanie Klein and critical social theory: An Account of politics, art, and reason based on her psychoanalytic theory*. New Haven, CT: Yale University Press.

Alford, C. F. (2009). *The Holocaust is not traumatic: The Holocaust can be represented*. Presented at the Annual Meeting of the Political Science Association, Toronto, Canada.

American Psychiatric Association. (2013). *Diagnostic and statistical manual of mental disorders (DSM-5)*. Washington, DC: Author.

Banyard, V. L., Moynihan, M. M., & Plante, E. G. (2007). Sexual violence prevention through bystander education: An experimental evaluation. *Journal of Community Psychology, 35*(4), 463–481. https://doi.org/10.1002/jcop.20159

Bart, P. B., & O'Brian, P. (1985). *Stopping rape: Successful survival strategies*. New York, NY: Teachers College Press.

Benjamin, J. (2018). *Beyond doer and done to* (1st ed.). New York, NY: Routledge.

Binswanger, O. (1922). Die kriegshysterie. In K. Bonhoeffer (Ed.), *Geistes-und nervenkrankheiten* (pp. 45–68). Leipzig, Germany: Johann Ambrosius Barth.

Bohmer, C., & Shuman, A. (2008). *Rejecting refugees: Political asylum in the 21st century*. London, UK: Routledge.

Breslau, J. (2004). Introduction: Cultures of trauma: Anthropological views of post-traumatic stress disorder in international health. *Culture, Medicine and Psychiatry, 28*(2), 113–126. https://doi.org/10.1023/B:MEDI.0000034421.07612.c8

Brown, W. B. (2008). Another emerging "storm": Iraq and Afghanistan veterans with PTSD in the criminal justice system. *Justice Policy Journal, 5*(2), 1–37.

Brownmiller, S. (1975). *Against our will: Men, women and rape.* New York, NY: Fawcett Books.

Bruner, J., & Lucariello, J. (1989). Monologue as narrative recreation of the world. In K. Nelson (Ed.), *Narratives from the crib* (pp. 73–97). Cambridge, MA: Harvard University Press.

Burack, C. (2002). IV. Re-Kleining Feminist Psychoanalysis. *Feminism & Psychology, 12*(1), 33–38.

California Innocence Project. (2019). *Parole.* Retrieved April 23, 2019, from California Innocence Project website: https://californiainnocenceproject.org/issues-we-face/parole/

Caruth, C. (2014). *Listening to trauma: Conversations with leaders in the theory and treatment of catastrophic experience.* Baltimore, MD: John Hopkins University Press.

Castelloe, M. (2019). *Vamik's room* [Documentary]. Retrieved from www.vamiksroom.org

Collins, P. H. (2000). *Black feminist thought: Knowledge, consciousness, and the politics of empowerment* (2nd ed.). New York, NY: Routledge.

Cortright, D. (1975). *Soldiers in revolt: GI resistance during the Vietnam War.* Chicago, IL: Haymarket Books.

Crenshaw, K. (1991). Mapping the margins: Intersectionality, identity politics, and violence against women of color. *Stanford Law Review, 43*(6), 1241–1299. https://doi.org/10.2307/1229039

Crenshaw, K. (1992). Race, gender, and sexual harassment. *Southern California Law Review, 65*, 1467–1476.

Dadlez, E. M., & Andrews, W. L. (2010). Post-abortion syndrome: Creating an affliction. *Bioethics, 24*(9), 445–452. https://doi.org/10.1111/j.1467-8519.2009.01739.x

Echterhoff, G., & Hirst, W. (2009). Social influence on memory. *Social Psychology, 40*(3), 106–110. Retrieved from http://econtent.hogrefe.com/doi/abs/10.1027/1864-9335.40.3.106

Fassin, D. (2012). *Humanitarian reason: A moral history of the present times.* Berkeley, CA: University of California Press.

Fassin, D., & Rechtman, R. (2009). *The empire of trauma: An inquiry into the condition of victimhood.* Princeton, NJ: Princeton University Press.

Frequently Asked Questions about Moral Injury. (n.d.). Retrieved December 19, 2019, from The Shay Moral Injury Center at Volunteers of America website: www.voa.org/moral-injury-center/moral-injury-faqs

Frueh, B. C., Hamner, M. B., Cahill, S. P., Gold, P. B., & Hamlin, K. L. (2000). Apparent symptom overreporting in combat veterans evaluated for PTSD. *Clinical Psychology Review, 20*(7), 853–885. https://doi.org/10.1016/S0272-7358(99)00015-X

Gentile, K. (October, 2015). *Chasing a justice-to-come: Sexual misconduct and boundary violations in the contexts of college campuses and psychoanalytic institutes.* Paper presented at the meetings of the Association for Psychoanalysis, Culture and Society, New Brunswick, NJ.

Gone, J. P. (2014). Reconsidering American Indian historical trauma: Lessons from an early Gros Ventre war narrative. *Transcultural Psychiatry, 51*(3), 387–406. https://doi.org/10.1177/1363461513489722

Green, H. H. (2019, November 14). *Rape survivors seeking asylum have to prove the rape happened or be deported—VICE* [News]. Retrieved December 20, 2019, from Vice News website: www.vice.com/en_us/article/d3aqez/trump-is-making-it-even-harder-for-rape-survivors-to-be-granted-asylum-us-puts-rape-survivors-on-trial

Griggs, R. A., & Whitehead, G. I. (2015). Coverage of Milgram's obedience experiments in social psychology textbooks: Where have all the criticisms gone? *Teaching of Psychology, 42*(4), 315–322. https://doi.org/10.1177/0098628315603065

Grossman, D. (2009). *On killing: The psychological cost of learning to kill in war and society* (Revised edition). New York, NY: Back Bay Books.

Haaken, J. (1998). *Pillar of salt: Gender, memory, and the perils of looking back.* New Brunswick, NJ: Rutgers University Press.

Haaken, J. (2002a). Bitch and femme psychology: Women, aggression, and psychoanalytic social theory. *Journal for the Psychoanalysis of Culture & Society, 7*(2), 202–215.

Haaken, J. (2002b). Cultural amnesia: Memory, trauma, and war. *Signs: Journal of Women in Culture and Society, 28*(1), 455–457. https://doi.org/10.1086/340870

Haaken, J. (2008a). Too close for comfort: Psychoanalytic cultural theory and domestic violence politics. *Psychoanalysis, Culture & Society, 13*(1), 75–93. https://doi.org/10.1057/palgrave.pcs.2100150

Haaken, J. (2008b). When White Buffalo Calf Woman meets Oedipus on the road: Lakota psychology, feminist psychoanalysis, and male violence. *Theory & Psychology, 18*(2), 195–208. https://doi.org/10.1177/0959354307087881

Haaken, J. (2010). *Hard knocks: Domestic violence and the psychology of storytelling.* New York, NY: Routledge.

Haaken, J. (2016). Riding the waves of feminism: Psychoanalysis and women's liberation. *Psychoanalysis, Culture & Society, 21*(3), 223–231. https://doi.org/10.1057/pcs.2016.5

Haaken, J. (2017). Many mornings after: Campus sexual assault and feminist politics. *Family Relations, 66*(1), 17–28. https://doi.org/10.1111/fare.12227

Haaken, J. (2018). Vamik's room [Review of the documentary film Vamik's Room, 2019]. *Psychoanalysis, Culture & Society, 23*(4), 480–484. https://doi.org/10.1057/s41282-018-0109-9

Haaken, J., & Heymann, C. (2005). *Diamonds, guns, and rice [Documentary]* [Documentary]. Ooligan Press.

Haaken, J., Ladum, A., Tarr, S. de, Zundel, K., & Heymann, C. (2005). *Speaking out: Women, war and the global economy.* Portland, OR: Ooligan Press.

Haaken, J., & O'Neill, M. (2014). Moving images: Psychoanalytically informed visual methods in documenting the lives of women migrants and asylum seekers. *Journal of Health Psychology, 19*(1), 79–89. https://doi.org/10.1177/1359105313500248

Haaken, J., & Palmer, T. (2012). War stories: Discursive strategies in framing military sexual trauma. *Psychoanalysis, Culture & Society, 17*(3), 325–333. https://doi.org/10.1057/pcs.2012.7

Haaken, J., Wallin-Ruschman, J., & Patange, S. (2012). Global hip-hop identities: Black youth, psychoanalytic action research, and the Moving to the Beat project. *Journal of Community & Applied Social Psychology, 22*(1), 63–74. https://doi.org/10.1002/casp.1097

Herman, J. (2017, November 26). *Out of the ashes: An interview with Judith Herman* (D. Jensen, Interviewer) [Internet]. Retrieved from https://dgrnewsservice.org/civilization/alienation/ashes-interview-judith-herman/

hooks, b. (1982). *Ain't I a woman: Black women and feminism.* London, UK: Pluto Press.

James, E. C. (2004). The political economy of "trauma" in Haiti in the democratic era of insecurity. *Culture, Medicine and Psychiatry, 28*(2), 127–149. https://doi.org/10.1023/B:MEDI.0000034407.39471.d4

Kang, H. K., & Bullman, T. A. (1996). Mortality among U.S. veterans of the Persian Gulf War. *The New England Journal of Medicine, 335*(20), 1498–1504. https://doi. org/10.1056/NEJM199611143352006

Kime, P. (2016, February 11). *Panel to VA: Stop studying causes of Gulf War illnesses, focus on treatment* [News]. Retrieved December 19, 2019, from Military Times website: www.militarytimes.com/pay-benefits/military-benefits/health-care/2016/02/11/panel-to-va-stop-studying-causes-of-gulf-war-illnesses-focus-on-treatment/

Kintsch, W., & Greene, E. (1978). The role of culture-specific schemata in the comprehension and recall of stories. *Discourse Processes, 1*(1), 1–13. https://doi. org/10.1080/01638537809544425

Kinzie, J. D., Manson, S. M., Vinh, D. T., Tolan, N. T., Anh, B., & Pho, T. N. (1982). Development and validation of a Vietnamese-language depression rating scale. *The American Journal of Psychiatry, 139*(10), 1276–1281. https://doi.org/10.1176/ajp.139.10.1276

Kleinman, A. (2012). Rebalancing academic psychiatry: Why it needs to happen—and soon. *The British Journal of Psychiatry, 201*(6), 421–422. http://dx.doi.org.proxy.lib. pdx.edu/10.1192/bjp.bp.112.118695

Laing, R. D. (1967). The Politics of Experience. New York. *Pantheon, 19.*

Latané, B., & Darley, J. M. (1970). *The unresponsive bystander: Why doesn't he help?* New York, NY: Appleton-Century-Crofts.

Levin, S. (2017, February 11). Army veterans return to Standing Rock to form a human shield against police. *The Guardian.* Retrieved from www.theguardian.com/us-news/2017/feb/11/standing-rock-army-veterans-camp

Loftus, E., & Ketcham, K. (1996). *The myth of repressed memory: False memories and allegations of sexual abuse* (Revised). New York, NY: St. Martin's Griffin.

Marcus, S. (2002). Fighting bodies, fighting words: A theory and politics of rape prevention. In J. Butler & J. W. Scott (Eds.), *Feminists theorize the political* (pp. 385–403). New York, NY: Routledge.

McMahon, S., Peterson, N. A., Winter, S. C., Palmer, J. E., Postmus, J. L., & Koenick, R. A. (2015). Predicting bystander behavior to prevent sexual assault on college campuses: The role of self-efficacy and intent. *American Journal of Community Psychology, 56*, 46–56. https://doi.org/10.1007/s10464-015-9740-0

McNally, R. J. (2003). Progress and controversy in the study of posttraumatic stress disorder. *Annual Review of Psychology, 54*, 229–252. https://doi.org/10.1146/annurev. psych.54.101601.145112

McNally, R. J. (2009). Can we fix PTSD in DSM-V? *Depression and Anxiety, 26*(7), 597–600. https://doi.org/10.1002/da.20586

Mollica, R. F., Caspi-Yavin, Y., Bollini, P., Truong, T., Tor, S., & Lavelle, J. (1992). The Harvard Trauma Questionnaire: Validating a cross-cultural instrument for measuring torture, trauma, and posttraumatic stress disorder in Indochinese refugees. *Journal of Nervous and Mental Disease, 180*(2), 111–116. https://doi.org/10.1097/00005053-199202000-00008

Mollica, R. F., Wyshak, G., de Marneffe, D., Khuon, F., & Lavelle, J. (1987). Indochinese versions of the Hopkins Symptom Checklist-25: A screening instrument for the psychiatric care of refugees. *The American Journal of Psychiatry, 144*(4), 497–500. https://doi.org/10.1176/ajp.144.4.497

Nash, W. P., & Litz, B. T. (2013). Moral injury: A mechanism for war-related psychological trauma in military family members. *Clinical Child and Family Psychology Review, 16*(4), 365–375.

O'Neill, M. (2010). *Asylum, migration and community.* Bristol, UK: Policy Press.

Paratore, L. (2016). "Insight" into life crimes: The rhetoric of remorse and rehabilitation in California parole precedent and practice. *Berkley Journal of Criminal Law*, *21*(1), 95–125.

Pecora, P. J., White, C. R., Jackson, L. J., & Wiggins, T. (2009). Mental health of current and former recipients of foster care: A review of recent studies in the USA. *Child & Family Social Work*, *14*(2), 132–146. https://doi.org/10.1111/j.1365-2206.2009.00618.x

Pupavac, V. (2004). War on the couch: The emotionology of the new international security paradigm. *European Journal of Social Theory*, *7*(2), 149–170. https://doi.org/10.1177/1368431004041749

Rentschler, C. A. (2011). *Second wounds: Victims' rights and the media in the U.S.* Durham, NC: Duke University Press.

Shatan, C. (1989). Happiness is a warm gun: Militarized mourning and ceremonial vengeance. *Vietnam Generation*, *1*(3), 127–151. Retrieved from https://digitalcommons.lasalle.edu/cgi/viewcontent.cgi?article=1036&context=vietnamgeneration

Shay, J. (1994). *Achilles in Vietnam: Combat trauma and the undoing of character*. New York, NY: Simon and Schuster.

Spence, D. P. (2001). The life history method applied to the refugee context. In W. Jeon, M. Yoshioka, & R. F. Mollica (Eds.), *Science of refugee mental health: New concepts and methods*. Tualatin, OR: Human Services Research Institute.

Spitzer, R. L., First, M. B., & Wakefield, J. C. (2007). Saving PTSD from itself in DSM-V. *Journal of Anxiety Disorders*, *21*(2), 233–241. Retrieved from www.beforeyoutakethatpill.com/2009/3/spitzer.pdf

Sturken, M. (1997). *Tangled memories: The Vietnam War, the AIDS epidemic, and the politics of remembering*. Berkeley, CA: University of California Press.

Summerfield, D. (1999). A critique of seven assumptions behind psychological trauma programmes in war-affected areas. *Social Science & Medicine*, *48*(10), 1449–1462. https://doi.org/10.1016/S0277-9536(98)00450-X

Tangney, J. P., Stuewig, J., & Hafez, L. (2011). Shame, guilt and remorse: Implications for offender populations. *The Journal of Forensic Psychiatry & Psychology*, *22*(5), 706–723. https://doi.org/10.1080/14789949.2011.617541

Volkan, V. D. (1998). Ethnicity and nationalism: A psychoanalytic perspective. *Applied Psychology*, *47*(1), 45–57. https://doi.org/10.1111/j.1464-0597.1998.tb00012.x

Volkan, V. D. (1999). Psychoanalysis and diplomacy: Part I. Individual and large group identity. *Journal of Applied Psychoanalytic Studies*, *1*(1), 29–55. https://doi.org/10.1023/A:1023026107157

Volkan, V. D. (2001). Transgenerational transmissions and chosen traumas: An aspect of large-group identity. *Group Analysis*, *34*(1), 79–97. https://doi.org/10.1177/05333160122077730

Yefet, K. C. (2016). Feminism and hyper-masculinity in Israel: A case study in deconstructing legal fatherhood. *Yale Journal of Law and Feminism*, *27*(1), 47–94.

# Conclusions

After interviewing Major Jim Sardo for the *Mind Zone* documentary, something he said stuck in my mind. A psychologist and Army reservist deployed twice to Iraq, Sardo was deeply familiar with psychiatric symptoms associated with war zones. "Most soldiers do not develop full-blown post-traumatic stress disorder," he explained, "but they may experience *pieces* of the disorder. They may find that they are more depressed than they were before, or that they are more anxious than before." In this book, I have tried to gather up pieces of the posttraumatic stress disorder phenomenon to understand what those pieces say about the profession of psychiatry itself. The assigning of this diagnosis, like any diagnosis, follows procedural rules for inclusion and exclusion of symptoms. One theme of the book centers on how the progressive reach of the diagnosis falls short of its grasp and how a vast landscape of human distress disappears from psychiatric view. Many of the cases taken up here follow psychiatry into war zones—those sites most highly associated with the development of PTSD. But I show how these war zones create more than just military trauma. They also produce forms of psychiatric knowledge and expertise that, much like other military technologies, are carried into the management of broader social anxieties and cultural crises.

In the Introduction, I describe PTSD as a diagnosis that grew out of the union of studies in *stress* and *trauma*. For over a century, the United States government and private industry have supported research on human responses to stress. The Yerkes–Dodson law—perhaps the closest phenomenon we have to a natural law in psychology—grew out of military research on stress during World War I. The law can be demonstrated in a wide range of animals and settings and is represented as an inverted-U curve: As stress on an organism increases, performance rises until a threshold is crossed where performance declines or breaks down. For over a century, industry and the military have attempted to pin down on research graphs the points of optimal stress before breaking down. Trauma can be conceptualized along the Yerkes–Dodson curve as that slope where adaptive capacities fail in the face of the magnitude of a stressor. Research on PTSD draws on the quantitative orientation of many stress studies, but the field also enlists narrative conventions in the trauma field—the idea of a dramatic rupture in the psyche. Trauma invites modes of storytelling that situate the rupture within a moral community of responsibility for suffering.

While the condition found an important place in folk diagnoses of maladies of modern life, PTSD appeals through its association with a dramatic rupture in states of normalcy. Enlisted as a lay diagnosis of acute distress, PTSD registers how impacts can linger beyond an initial state of crisis. But my analysis of this diagnosis centers on how it migrates in the field of psychiatry in response to psychiatry's own crisis of legitimacy.

A set of questions from my field research informs this study of posttraumatic stress disorder. One centers on the relative progressiveness of the PTSD diagnosis—and whether its use in the many institutional settings where it is invoked contributes to campaigns for social justice. The expansion of the PTSD diagnosis both signaled and silenced a widening range of political grievances. I return to the union of stress and trauma studies, and to how chronic hardship and stress conditions lost ground to the more riveting scenes associated with trauma. A second line of analysis enlists critical traditions in the anti-psychiatry movement to address the dilemmas documented throughout the book. If PTSD is in part symptomatic of a crisis in the field of psychiatry, how might we think differently about the role of psychiatry in responding to socially produced suffering? A third question looks at the role of psychoanalysis in the PTSD movement, including social interventions where psychoanalysis has played a leading role but has struggled for scientific legitimacy within the framework of the medical model. In my Conclusions, I return to these recurring questions and themes, and to crisis settings where clinicians are caught in some of the same forms of institutional madness as those confronted by people under their care. In this Conclusions chapter, I return to these recurring questions and themes.

## Is PTSD a Progressive Diagnosis?

A decade after PTSD was ushered into the DSM-III, legal scholar Alan Stone (1993) waxed rhapsodic over its historical significance. "No diagnosis in the history of American psychiatry has had a more dramatic and pervasive impact on law and social justice than post-traumatic stress disorder." He adds that its scientific acceptance in psychiatry "has given a new credibility to a variety of victims who come before the courts either as defendants or plaintiffs" (p. 23). PTSD has found its place in the legal tools available for attorneys and thus represents one kind of progressive advance in the use of psychiatric expertise. But it's important to assess as well the costs of those legal victories.

The early PTSD movement indicted psychiatry as a profession deeply implicated in human suffering, from over-pathologizing and over-medicating in response to patients' complaints to its failure to address societal sources of mental disturbances. Many critical psychologists enlist the concept of the "psy-complex" in diagnosing the pathologies of the professions. Parker (2015), Critical psychiatrist David Ingleby (1985), and social theorist Nikolas Rose (1985) developed the idiom of psy-complex to describe a system of ideas and professional practices that accompanied the emergence in the 19th century of psychology, psychiatry, medicine, and criminology—disciplines critical to the production of ideas about normalcy and deviancy. In an early work provocatively titled *The Psychological Complex*, Rose (1985) makes use of the psychodynamic notion of mental complexes (e.g., Oedipal, inferiority, guilt, God complex) to map the disturbances of the professions and their roles in the ideology and governance of modern societies. Parker enlists this line of analysis to critique assessment tools and psychiatric treatments oriented toward personal adjustment. He offers that critical psychology is "an attempt to problematize the place of psychological explanations in patterns of power and ideology . . . and particularly with reference to questions of what is normal and abnormal" (2014, p. 6).

Given this wider critique of diagnosis and the medical model, why focus on PTSD? Aren't other disorders equally implicated in this psy-complex? My interest in PTSD is guided by its position as a political response to campaigns by progressive clinicians to address societal sources of many mental disorders. Prior to the PTSD movement, there were diagnoses that included situational factors in their criteria such as *adjustment disorder* and *stress reaction*. But these conditions were thought to be of a limited duration. The dominant thinking in psychiatry for over a century was that normal people return to base-line functioning within weeks or months following exposure to a traumatic event. PTSD brought the politics of psychopathology directly into the clinical picture.

The PTSD diagnosis was formulated in the context of the Vietnam War and influenced by the work of Robert Jay Lifton and others who argued that American soldiers who carried out atrocities in Vietnam were actually victims of US foreign policy and to crisis settings where clinicians are caught in some of the same forms of institutional madness as are those confronted by people under their care. In reflecting on this debate over whether veterans were victims or perpetrators, Peter Marin (1981) suggests that therapists in this early movement saw their jobs as helping veterans with their post-war adjustment. As a college instructor who led groups of Vietnam veterans, Marin concludes that what many veterans suffered from was "profound moral distress that may defy therapy" (Marin, 1981, p. 68). Marin charges that much of the stress literature and the treatment approaches at the time tend to "empty the vets' experience of moral content, to defuse and bowdlerize it" (p. 72).

One way of thinking about the progressiveness of a diagnosis is in its capacity to hold the complexity of the symptoms and the human dilemmas that give rise to them. As Jessica Benjamin (2018) concludes, working with trauma requires moving beyond the simple dichotomy of "doer and done to." The PTSD diagnosis fares poorly in the criminal justice system, however, where cases fail to conform to conventional notions of virtuous victimhood. Indeed, even when the diagnosis is used in cases where battered women kill their partners, PTSD has not persuaded juries in "atypical cases"—those cases where the woman exhibits anger or animus toward her abuser. It has been more effective in cases where women are cast as passive victims overtaken by rage in a dissociated state (Berger et al., 2012; Sparr, 2007).

The burgeoning literature on *moral injury* similarly locates the source of harms in an external agency. Moral injury provides a corrective to PTSD in extending the syndrome beyond psycho-physiological responses into what advocates term "wounds of the soul." But in capturing some of the disturbing remainder of what prototypical PTSD leaves behind, the moral injury concept reproduces the medico-forensic impact model of trauma and obscures the larger terrain of moral responsibility, including situations where victims may be implicated in some way. In talking with Vietnam veterans groups, Marin (1981) called for a social redistribution of responsibility for the war. "Yes the vets were guilty, but many of us [the public] had been guilty also," he reports of a conversation with a defensive veteran. But he shifts the load of guilt from the shoulders of individual vets to the larger American public, adding that "we were guilty not only for the war but for countless public and private acts whose consequences had been pain or suffering for others" (p. 77).

There is risk in such calls for a diffusion of responsibility as well. If all are responsible, then no one is specifically responsible. For decades, feminists have been wary of psychological interventions that humanize male perpetrators, although many Black and Indigenous feminists emphasize moving beyond simple victim/perpetrator categories. In settings where perpetrators of crimes are also victims, including victims of institutional forms of trauma, campaigns to enlist the PTSD diagnosis in their defense have failed for the most part because the category is itself an externalizing strategy. In a society that hyper-individualizes responsibility for personal problems, PTSD offers some salutary relief. Even when it delivers material benefits, however, the diagnosis does strip accounts of moral complexity.

In interviewing psychiatrists and patients at the Oregon State Hospital, I was struck by how many personal incidents of trauma were reported in patients' medical records and yet how few of them were officially diagnosed with PTSD. Rather, the diagnosis circulated among staff members as an informal expression of sympathy. State statutes disallow personality disorder diagnoses for state hospitals, but PTSD also fares poorly because it positions the person as a victim. Patients gain entry as victims of their *own mental illness*—a condition of the person that compromises moral capacities. Many of the patients were hospitalized under the insanity plea, and some as part of the adjudication of murder or attempted murder.

As psychologist Alex Millkey explained, most people who kill someone do not go on to commit another crime, partly because killing someone is traumatic for most people. Nonetheless, the accused—those defined as perpetrators—face a higher threshold in summoning public sympathies. One of those accused and hospitalized under the insanity plea was Tino—a Latino man who I interviewed five or six times in the course of filming *Guilty Except for Insanity*. Tino had been arrested for attempted murder of his boss. After falling from a roof on a construction site where he was working, Tino had picked up his hammer and assaulted his boss who was subsequently hospitalized with severe injuries. Tino was charged with attempted murder. In reading the police report,

I noticed that the officers had interviewed several co-workers who were on the job site. They told the police that Tino had been harassed for some time by other co-workers and subjected to racial slurs. There also were questions about safety and pressures on workers that may have contributed to Tino falling off the roof. But the violence of his reaction when he hit the ground required a psychiatric assessment. He described his own state as dissociated and claimed that he had no memory of the assault nor why he had attacked his boss.

Tino was evaluated at the state hospital and diagnosed as suffering from a psychotic disorder not otherwise specified (NOS). One area of symptoms centered on what his psychiatrist described as Tino's "excessive preoccupation with numbers and codes." When he was evaluated in jail, Tino was observed spending much of his time writing on his court papers. He filled the sheets with elaborate formulas and dates accompanied by what appeared to be random numbers and letters. He held these papers tightly in his possession as he was shuttled over several years between the jail, the hospital for evaluation, to court and back to jail, and then finally committed under the insanity defense.

When I asked Tino to tell me about the formulas he wrote on his court papers, he said that the only possessions he was allowed in jail were these court documents explaining why he was there. He described how he kept his mind busy by remembering various dates and creating a code for memories connected to those dates. It struck me that Tino and his psychiatrist were caught in the same system of madness: The psychiatrist was required to navigate the state legal statutes and *Diagnostic and Statistical Manual*, each of which encompassed mind-numbing lists of numbered categories and abbreviated references to state laws, and Tino generated his own code for navigating this same world. When he showed me his court document with its typed legalese and his own fastidiously written codes filling every space and margin, I thought to myself, "this looks pretty crazy." But I also thought, "this is his way of holding onto himself in a crazy system." Critical psychologists would add that this document was itself a commentary on the madness of the psy-complex. This psychiatrist was known by many patients—including Tino—to be quite compassionate. He often defended Tino before the Psychiatric Security Board as not a danger to the public and testified that it was not really clear what happened on the day of the crime. But the rationality of the doctor's numbers and codes won out over those generated by Tino because the doctor's signs were part of a larger chain of signifiers. Tino's signs were idiosyncratic and failed to communicate rationality.

One progressive intervention of the PTSD movement was in challenging conventional legal rules centered on assumed proximity of a causal event and symptoms in response to that event. A contentious legal debate unfolded around psychiatric explanations for temporal delays between an event such as a military attack on the combat unit and unlawful behavior (Sparr, 2007). The longer the delay between the event and the crime, the less likely juries are to be sympathetic. These delays are more apt to tip judicial assessments into the personality disorder categories, as lapses in time suggest cunningly willful or criminal intent.

The strategy of delayed memory—the claim that PTSD symptoms could surface years or decades after exposure to trauma—carried problematic freight over time, however, as accounts confronted forensic metrics for evaluating their veracity. In the anti-war speak-outs of the early 1970s, the truth of the story was in its collective validity. Early PTSD advocates enlisted veterans' nightmarish flashbacks to make the case against war. But by the 1980s, trauma diagnoses emerged as a new frontier in broader cultural wars. Mental health advocates pointed out how people living on the streets exhibited symptoms much like soldiers returning from war zones. Yet for so many people living under police state conditions or struggling with the soul-crushing stresses of poverty, meeting Criterion A—producing the index trauma story—was nearly impossible. The PTSD diagnosis required a temporally located event. The social symbolic power of delayed memory, the idea that veterans carried the societally forgotten effects of warfare through their clinical complaints, confronted evidentiary rules in courts that bar these more elusive dynamics of the clinical picture. Advocates won recognition for PTSD within a narrow medico-legal framework that requires literal facts and individualized accounts separated from the collective lamentations that gave rise to them.

The clinical validity of the PTSD diagnosis required that the "extreme stressor" criterion departed from everyday experience. Even though everyone theoretically could develop PTSD as a "normal response to an abnormal situation," the claims of oppressed groups, including the poor and the incarcerated, were a poor fit for the prototype. The progressive reach of the diagnosis confronted the limits of its grasp. A new campaign arose to bridge the gap, one that failed to gain DSM support—a campaign to recognize complex posttraumatic stress disorder (CPTSD) as a clinical diagnosis. While chronic forms of PTSD were recognized in terms of enduring symptoms, the DSM committees hold to a strict boundary between reactions for which there was a discreet cause and the more pervasive forms of suffering that can produce many of the same symptoms. The diagnosis required a dramatic story with a clear beginning, middle, and ending.

## Toward a Progressive Psychiatry

The anti-psychiatry movement of the 1960s and 1970s differed from mainstream psychiatry in approaching psychiatric symptoms as meaningful communications and in interrogating conventional notions of normalcy. Those expressing signs of schizophrenia or other major disturbances had something to say about society and the human condition. The campaign to recognize PTSD did signal a new era of revolt against medical psychiatry and a revival of currents of the anti-psychiatry movement. Trauma symptoms were cast as registers of cultural amnesia—of societally forgotten abuses that live on in the psyches of survivors. Unlike the anti-psychiatry movement, however, the PTSD movement's struggle with psychiatry centered on securing passage for this disorder into the medical taxonomy and fighting for its legitimacy within the DSM system.

Revisiting touchstone ideas in the anti-psychiatry tradition—also termed critical psychiatry—provides a pathway into thinking about the progressiveness of the PTSD diagnosis. Termed "alienists" in the 19th century, psychiatrists assumed positions of medical authority within the asylum system and its disciplinary regime. As psychoanalyst Thomas Szasz (1995) describes this history, the psychiatrist was sought out by people who were invested in managing others, often a troublesome family member. From the start, asylum psychiatrists were charged with social and political control of behavior. It was not until the late 19th century that psychiatry emerged from the shadows of the asylum and secured legitimacy as a medical science (Misbach & Stam, 2006). For Szasz, the "myth of mental illness" was in its scientific disguise, its reliance on a disease model to rationalize institutional coercion and control. He was correct in the sense that mental disorders are not illnesses in the ordinary medical sense. But as Ian Parker (2014) points out, Szasz's libertarian stance "throws people back to the wolves in the market-place, rather than doing something to help them" (p. 11).

Szasz and Michel Foucault are part of a philosophical tradition that challenges the progressive narrative of psychiatry, although their critiques point to very different notions of progress (Bracken & Thomas, 2010 Haaken, 2015). Szasz situates psychiatry as a transfer of power within secular modernity. Doctors secured authority as agents of the state to confine a person not charged with crimes but otherwise bothersome, "rendering him childlike, and justifying controlling and caring for him against his will" (Szasz, 1995, p. 2). This critique of psychiatry took hold during the de-institutionalization movement of the 1960s amid campaigns to limit forced confinement of persons, including holding people for purposes of evaluation. The history of psychiatry told by Foucault (2006) brings some of these same elements of rationalized control into the critical analysis. He traces the history of mechanical restraints used in asylums, for example, and how these methods had little to do with the scientific discourses circulating at the time. Foucault argues that the rise of institutions charged with care of "imbeciles and idiots" required raising funds to support the institution. In order to rationalize need for subsidies, psychiatrists were forced to exaggerate their medical reports to "depict the idiot or mental defective as someone who is dangerous" (p. 220). But for Foucault, these displays of psychiatric authority reflect a deeper problem at the heart of modernity: the reliance of modern states on experts and scientific taxonomies. Power in this context is not simply a constraining force, as Szasz would suggest, nor is it best understood as holding back the free rein of human nature. Foucault places psychiatry in the context of discursive practices—systems of ideas for organizing knowledge.

For Foucault, psychiatry operates as a modern form of expertise because it produces typologies and systems of thought that shape everyday thinking about mental life.

Foucault holds some affinity with Freud in their mutual skepticism toward the Enlightenment project—the 18th-century European movement centered on a vision of progress organized around rational control over nature, including human nature. From a Foucauldian perspective, a critical psychiatry works to decenter the authority of psychiatric discourse by exposing its own historical contingencies. In *Madness and Civilization*, Foucault identifies with the anti-psychiatry movement in calling for subversive discursive practices: "they are the discourses of the madman, the patient, the delinquent, the pervert and other persons who, in their respective times, held knowledges about themselves which diverged from the established categories" (Foucault, 1965, p 16).

As a theorist and practitioner aligned with the anti-psychiatry movement of the 1970s, Peter Sedgwick (1982) argues that the real issue in psychiatry involves the relationship of psychiatric institutions to the larger society and public responsibilities to people who are disturbed. He argues that anti-psychiatry can perpetuate suffering through its own grandiose campaigns to liberate madness from the repressive hold of medicine. Further, the notion of mental illness, whether a myth or not, is used by countless people because it expresses their claims for some form of care. Whether cast as mentally ill or experiencing extreme states, those who have trouble functioning within established bounds of normalcy do have things to say that are worth hearing. But, as Sedgwick points out, romanticizing madness can be as oppressive as phobic avoidance. His analysis includes demands for community-based mental health services but extends into confronting public fears that contribute to the isolation and oppression of people who seem odd.

While schizophrenia took center stage as the prototypical form of madness in the anti-psychiatry movement, the PTSD campaign advanced by showing how normal people could look quite crazy under conditions of extreme stress. And there is something to this claim. But this campaign also marginalized those who fell outside the bounds of this conception of normalcy. The Hearing Voices movement of the early 21st-century carried some of Sedgwick's critical spirit into the mental health field. Sedgwick's critique of psychiatry centered on its tendency to isolate those identified as mentally ill and to strip them of their own complex subjectivity. Ian Parker (2014) extends this line of critique further in suggesting that

> a premise of social justice from the standpoint of those who are speaking for themselves is that we do not require them to speak the same language as us as a condition for being heard, and that we acknowledge that there is no common language for describing "madness" inside psychology.
>
> (p. 3)

I recall screening *Guilty Except for Insanity* at a Hearing Voices conference in 2010—a conference that included mental health professionals and *service users*—a term preferred over patients or clients by many in this movement. During the screening and in discussion afterwards, audience vocalizations were varied and included emotional eruptions that through my clinical ear could be diagnosed as loose associations, pressured speech, and auditory hallucinations. Some were on psychiatric medications, but many chose a path of learning to live with the cacophony of internal persecutors. There was also recognition of how the social world they inhabit could amplify or temper disturbing voices. Many of the service users had acquired a range of diagnoses over time, including PTSD. But none of those categories adequately explained their states of mind.

Complex PTSD would likely not have served them any better. While some PTSD proponents fight for expanding the scope of the disorder to include complex PTSD, or for widening criteria for inclusion of groups such as asylum seekers, foster youth, and the incarcerated, this vision of progress ultimately preserves the position of psychiatric experts as gatekeepers—and it reproduces a hierarchy of complaints separating those with dramatic tales from those accounts of hardship less apt to move institutional border guards.

PTSD emerged as a symptom in the field of psychiatry—a compromise formation that both acknowledges and disavows the long-term effects of societally produced stress and suffering. Its protean qualities as a diagnosis—its capacity to take many forms and encompass a broad range of non-specific effects—lends itself to migration across social borders and to recognition by the US military itself as part of the calculus of warfare. Although estimates of the risk for posttraumatic stress disorder among veterans vary widely, the risk is now factored into military planning as are combat stress control units in the management of its associated symptoms. Many of the military clinicians interviewed in the course of my field work expressed pride in the "new Army" and its shift from phobic avoidance and shaming of soldiers who break down in the course of military service to a more caring approach. From a Foucauldian perspective, we can recognize how the PTSD diagnosis has been incorporated into the rationalizing system of the modern psy-complex.

## Psychoanalysis and Trauma Disorders

A third line of argument in this book centers on the role of psychoanalysis in the history of trauma diagnoses and how psychoanalysis lost its critical potential as it joined forces to advance the posttraumatic stress disorder diagnosis. As a lay diagnosis invoked as folk commentary on suffering, PTSD foregrounds complaints that call for public supports and sympathies. The power of this relatively destigmatized label in everyday contexts is limited. But this book takes up settings where clinical procedures enter the picture though the accompanying authority of experts. In many of the historical cases and contexts explored in this book, psychoanalysis departs from medical psychiatry in widening the interpretive lens for diagnostic storytelling. It allows for ambiguity, for dynamic shifts in the meaning of events over time, and for the symbolic and metaphorical registers of symptoms. The dynamic unconscious refers less to a non-rational or primitive substrate of mind than to the human struggle to create coherence out of the fluctuating external and internal claims on consciousness and the object-seeking aspects of the mind itself.

In my own use of psychoanalytic traditions, I have been drawn more to the spatial metaphors of center and periphery than the topographical metaphors of early Freudian theory. This spatial frame orients observations to finding meaning in the periphery of what is most readily noticed. Here there is some affinity with Foucault who declares his critical project as not being one of uncovering hidden truths from under an ideological veil of deception. Rather, it is in attending to knowledge "located low on the hierarchy" and the "reappearance of this knowledge, of these local popular knowledges, these disqualified knowledges, that criticism performs its work" (as cited in Smart, 1994, p. 105). It is worth noting that it was in those eras when psychoanalysis lost its status in the field of psychiatry—the period of the 1970s when psychoanalysts were no longer the reigning authorities in major medical centers—that psychoanalysis came to flourish in the humanities and feminist studies.

Psychoanalysis has produced a rich history of clinical thinking about the complexities of psychic defenses and modes of representing overwhelming events. Psychological defenses such as denial, emotional numbing, obsessive reliving of events, and behavioral acting out have been observed for centuries. But expertise, including psychoanalytic expertise, requires the translation of field observations into theory and generalizable findings. Psychoanalysts have played leading roles in criminal court cases because of their skills in storytelling—a point developed in Chapter 2.

When psychoanalytic experts are deployed to war zones, however, they face the same pressures as other military clinicians to keep the war machine going. The ambiguity and metaphorical play with language that characterize psychoanalysis, its demands for patience before interpreting the story behind the symptom, collapses under the boot of the commanders. But Freud's interpretation of war neurosis is instructive in terms of the limits of psychoanalytic formulations as correctives to military psychiatry and responses to the pathologies of warfare. He explained how bodily paralysis—losing control of an arm so the soldier was no longer able to take up his weapon and fight—served as a compromise formation in escaping the conflict between military commands and the dictates of conscience. As long as the conflicts that gave rise to the conversion hysteria remained unconscious, psychoanalysis operated as a protective strategy. The symptom told an unconscious story of resistance. But once the conflict enters consciousness, the soldier confronts the full disciplinary force of the military.

Psychoanalysis operates oppressively when trauma diagnoses displace the political and social contexts of problems in conflict zones. To classify marginalized or persecuted groups as suffering from psychic trauma, even under the redemptive banner of PTSD, can foreclose on victims' own mode of framing their hardships. Whether assigned by a forensic team or psychiatric assessors, trauma marks individuals and groups in ways that they may choose not to be marked. Their dramatic stories of suffering may take center stage at the cost of recognizing their strategies of survival and solidarity.

Stephen Frosh (2007) points out that one can go too far with the idea of complexity and discursive unpacking of the manifold meanings of clinical material. As Donald Winnicott (1960) might frame the problem, clinicians must settle on "good-enough" interpretations. Clinicians working in crisis zones are confronted with intense institutional demands to intervene in situations where the problems elude the tools available to them. My interest here is in how collective and institutional defenses are embedded in rules for diagnostic storytelling and the costs of various strategies for administering relief.

One effect of this narrowing is in the hyper-individualizing of collective forms of suffering. Whether termed contagion effect or group hysteria, collective responses to distress tend to be either pathologized or cast outside the scope of observed mental health effects. Yet the group culture of male hysteria during World War I, like Charcot's displays of female hysteria in the late 19th century, offers an important site for thinking about the social registers of symptoms. The discovery during Charcot's era of the performative aspects of madness continues to hang over psychiatry as a shameful lesson in how doctors can be seduced by mesmerizing disorders. A critical psychoanalysis takes group dynamics into account and recognizes how shared identifications with a syndrome may communicate collective experiences of distress and forms of solidarity.

In commenting on the Truth and Reconciliation Commission (TRC) in Sierra Leone, Rosalind Shaw (2007) notes the hegemonic influence of Western psychoanalytic discourse on the confessional proceedings: "The truth that re-wounds but also cleanses, and upon which it is assumed that healing and reconciliation depend, is understood in terms of a painful verbalization of memories of violence." In commenting further on the hearings, she poses a question: "How did this understanding of truth-telling develop?" (p. 191). How do these particular speech acts acquire reparative currencies? Her response interrogates psychoanalysis as a Western import into TRC proceedings—one that depoliticizes collective suffering and frames reparation from war as a cathartic process. Converging with this psychiatric construction of post-war reparation, she adds, was the concept of "'post-traumatic stress disorder' and its treatment by verbal processing, which entails the painful narrative recapitulation of traumatic events from the past" (p. 192). In her telling of the denouement to TRC hearings, participants ultimately assess the confessionals in terms of the material supports provided by the government in redressing the aftermath of armed conflict. "If I get help, I'll forget about the war," Shaw cites one Sierra Leonean as observing, "but if you don't have help, you'll remember the war all the time" (p. 205).

The lessons Shaw draws from the Sierra Leonean TRC testimonials may be extended to survivors of conflicts in the global North as well. The PTSD movement created space for combat veterans and sexual abuse survivors to give voice to their grievances and to enlist psychiatry in the telling of their stories. Humans have evolved with physiological and psychological capacities to recover from losses, even from loss born of large-scale violence and trauma. But recovery depends on having the ground secure under your feet. Where social welfare and supports depend on establishing one's status as a worthy petitioner, the portal of entry into dignified assistance leaves many sufferers behind. The use of the PTSD diagnosis in disability claims registers the role of psychiatry in securing those portals of entry. The PTSD route reduces the complex and varied complaints of veterans even as it silences those not loud enough to register on the meters of audibility.

As we strolled by an encampment of people living on the streets one cold January morning, a colleague shared with me what felt to her to be a progressive insight. She explained that she had recently realized that many of the homeless people on the streets were actually veterans suffering from PTSD. They weren't just drug addicts or mentally ill people. The coupling of military service and trauma provided an optical aid, a means of acknowledging that people living outside have worth and value. They were people to be thanked for their service. It was like the gestalt double image of the vase and the face-to-face profiles. Looking at street people as veterans suffering the effects of PTSD allowed her to recognize their humanity. The idea enabled her to look without the distress of seeing. For the houseless veterans on the streets, my friend's invoking of this redemptive term seemed to echo the invitations at the airports for veterans to board the plane after the first-class passengers. But for many people living in those tents my friend and I passed, the dispossessed who struggle to survive on the mean streets of America every day, medical psychiatry offers even less in making their troubles visible.

## References

Benjamin, J. (2018). *Beyond doer and done to: Recognition theory, intersubjectivity and the third* (1st ed.). New York, NY: Routledge.

Berger, O., McNiel, D. E., & Binder, R. L. (2012). PTSD as a criminal defense: A review of case law. *Journal of the American Academy of Psychiatry and the Law*, *40*(4), 509–521.

Bracken, P., & Thomas, P. (2010). From Szasz to Foucault: On the role of critical psychiatry. *Philosophy, Psychiatry, & Psychology*, *17*(3), 219–228.

Foucault, M. (1965). *Madness and civilization: A history of insanity in the age of reason* (Vintage Books Edition and R. Howard, Trans.). New York, NY: Random House.

Foucault, M. (2006). *Psychiatric power: Lectures at the Collège de France, 1973–74* (J. Lagrange, F. Ewald, & A. Fontana, Eds. and G. Burchell, Trans.). New York, NY: Palgrave Macmillan.

Frosh, S. (2007). Disintegrating qualitative research. *Theory & Psychology, 17*(5), 635–653. https://doi.org/10.1177/0959354307081621

Haaken, J. (2015). Alienists and alienation. *Handbook of Critical Psychology, 213–221.*

Ingleby, D. (1985). Professionals and Socializers: The "Psy-complex". *Research in Law, Deviance and Control, 7:* 79–109.

Marin, P. (1981). Living in moral pain. *Psychology Today,* 71–80.

Miller, A. (2006). *The body never lies: The lingering effects of hurtful parenting* (Reprint edition and A. Jenkins, Trans.). New York, NY: W. W. Norton & Company.

Misbach, J., & Stam, H. J. (2006). Medicalizing melancholia: Exploring profiles of psychiatric professionalization. *Journal of the History of the Behavioral Sciences, 42*(1), 41–59. https://doi.org/10.1002/jhbs.20133

Parker, I. (2014). Madness and justice. *Journal of Theoretical and Philosophical Psychology, 34*(1), 28–40.

Parker, I. (Ed.). (2015). *Handbook of critical psychology.* New York, NY: Routledge.

Rose, N. (1985). *The psychological complex: Psychology, politics and society in England 1869–1939.* London, UK: Routledge & Kegan Paul.

Sedgwick, P. (1982). *Psycho politics: Laing, Foucault, Goffman, Szasz, and the future of mass psychiatry.* New York, NY: Harper & Row.

Shaw, R. (2007). Memory frictions: Localizing the Truth and Reconciliation Commission in Sierra Leone. *International Journal of Transitional Justice, 1*(2), 183–207. https://doi.org/10.1093/ijtj/ijm008

Smart, B. (Ed.). (1994). *Michel Foucault: Critical assessments: Vol. III.* New York, NY: Routledge.

Stone, A. A. (1993). Post-traumatic stress disorder and the law: Critical review of the new frontier. *Journal of the American Academy of Psychiatry and the Law Online, 21*(1), 23–36.

Sparr, L. F. (2007). Forensic issues associated with post-traumatic stress disorder: Twenty-five years later. In L. B. Schlesinger (Ed.), *Explorations in criminal psychopathology: Clinical syndromes with forensic implications* (2nd ed., pp. 297–327). Springfield, IL: Charles C. Thomas.

Szasz, T. (1995). The origin of psychiatry: The alienist as nanny for troublesome adults. *History of Psychiatry, 6*(21), 1–19. https://doi.org/10.1177/0957154X9500602101

van der Kolk, B. (2015). *The body keeps the score: Brain, mind, and body in the healing of trauma* (Reprint edition). New York, NY: Penguin Books.

Winnicott, D. W. (1960). The theory of the parent-infant relationship. *The International Journal of Psychoanalysis, 41,* 585–595. https://doi.org/10.1093/med:psych/9780190271381.003.0022

# Index

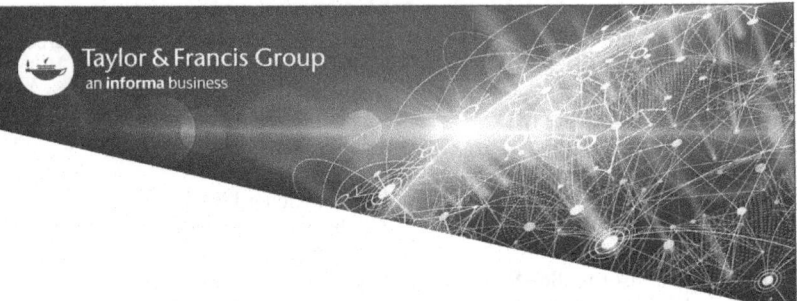
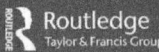
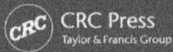